THE ELEMENTS OF HERBALISM

David L. Hoffmann has been practising as a consultant medical herbalist for many years, and has lectured widely on holistic herbalism, as well as personal and planetary transformation. He has also been active in the environmental movement, and has done much writing and broadcasting in these areas.

The *Elements Of* is a series designed to present high quality introductions to a broad range of essential subjects.

The books are commissioned specifically from experts in their fields. They provide readable and often unique views of the various topics covered, and are therefore of interest both to those who have some knowledge of the subject, as well as those who are approaching it for the first time.

Many of these concise yet comprehensive books have practical suggestions and exercises which allow personal experience as well as theoretical understanding, and offer a valuable source of information on many important themes.

In the same series

The Arthurian Tradition
Astrology
Buddhism
The Chakras
The Celtic Tradition
Christian Symbolism
Creation Myth
Dreamwork
The Goddess
The Grail Tradition
The Greek Tradition

Human Potential
Natural Magic
Pendulum Dowsing
Prophecy
Psychosynthesis
Ritual Magic
Shamanism
Sufism
Tai Chi
Visualisation

THE ELEMENTS OF

HERBALISM

David Hoffmann

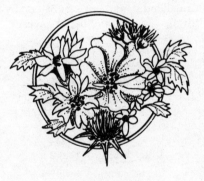

ELEMENT BOOKS

First published in Great Britain in 1990 by
Element Books Limited
Longmead, Shaftesbury, Dorset

Cover illustration by Miranda Gray
Cover design by Max Fairbrother
Typeset by Selectmove, London
Printed and bound in Great Britain by
Billings Ltd, Hylton Road, Worcester

British Library Cataloguing in Publication Data
Hoffmann, David 1951–
The elements of herbalism.
1. Medicine. Herbal remedies
I. Title
615.321

ISBN 1–85230–173–2

Thank you Diana,
for the Love with which you bless me,
and for being such an impeccable mid-wife as I gave birth to
this book.

We are part of the earth and it is part of us . . .
The earth does not belong to man; man belongs to the earth.
This we know.
All things are connected like the blood which unites one
family.

Chief Seattle

In all creation there are mysterious healing forces,
which no person can know unless they have been revealed
by God.
Hildegard Von Bingen, Book of Divine Works (*Liber
Divinorum Operum*)

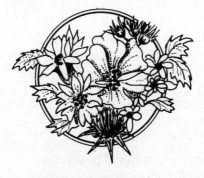

CONTENTS

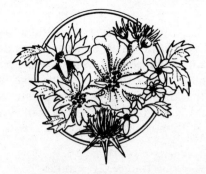

1 · HERBALISM – GAIA IN ACTION

Planet Earth – what a beautiful and bounteous world to call home. The more we turn our attention towards the nature of our relationship with the environment, the more profound become the insights into the close embrace we share. Whether on the global scale of our effects upon climate and the climate's effects upon us, or at the biochemical level of plants as medicines, the connections revealed are powerful and very real. Of the many ways in which our ecological inter-relatedness shows itself, the art and science of herbal medicine is for many people the most unexpected.

Above all else, herbalism is the medicine of belonging, the direct experience of the whole healing the part. Our world blesses us with herbs, with leaves of life. In the face of the blind abuse and rape of nature, we discover remedies that can help us survive the impact of humanity's mistakes. To heal ourselves we must know ourselves, and ecology, spirituality, intuition and common sense tell us that we are all one. If our world is sick and poisoned then so are we. If the forests are being destroyed, then we die a little with each felling. Every whale that is respected and allowed to live to blesses us. Each river cleaned and renewed flows through our veins and renews us.

Humanity is being faced with the realities of a shared planet. This may take the form of a drought caused by the Greenhouse Effect, pollution-induced birth defects or the purgatory of human overpopulation. On the other hand it may be the dawning recognition that the intimate embrace of our world is a healing force moving humanity towards a transformation of our relationship with the Earth, ourselves and each other.

THE GAIA HYPOTHESIS

The Gaia Hypothesis proposes an illuminating context within which to place herbs and humanity. First postulated by James Lovelock, it has been developed by many people, bridging the worlds of science and spirituality. Gaia was the Greek goddess of the Earth, consort of Uranus and mother of both the gods and the Titans. There are variations of spelling and pronunciation as the name is from Ancient Greece with its subtly different alphabet; Gaia, Gaea or Gæa are all used. Lovelock has suggested it as an appropriate name for the complex 'being' that is the whole of planet Earth. 'We have since defined Gaia as a complex entity involving the Earth's biosphere, atmosphere, oceans and soil; the totality constituting a feedback or cybernetic system which seeks an optimal physical and chemical environment for life on this planet.'[1]

Lovelock's research for NASA, investigating planetary biogeochemistry, led to his formulation of the Gaia Hypothesis, which suggests that the Earth is not a physico-chemical mechanism but a living entity with the equivalent of senses, intelligence, memory and the capacity to act. This is an entirely non-human intelligence that in our anthropocentric arrogance we do not directly perceive. Within the fabric of Gaia there is an interwoven and intelligently driven web which generates balance, continuity and stability. She is the Earth spirit, she is all things biological and inorganic, and she is also the interactions between them. She is ecology!

Formulation of the Gaia Hypothesis marks a special point in humanity's evolution. For the first time there is a clear point of contact between science and spirituality. Both world views can now agree that all of life is one, that the whole is more than the sum of the parts. This can be said in both mystical poetry or in terms of the physics of biogeochemistry, but the same thing is being expressed.

How does herbalism fit into this world view? Evolutionary biology tells us that all of a species's needs are met by its environment, otherwise it could not survive. This holds true for humanity as much as for slime moulds. The environment provides us not only with food, shelter and resources of all kinds, but also with waterfalls and the joy of sunsets. All human needs are met, spiritual as well as physical. Starvation and its associated evils are usually brought about by human blindness and greed. Whether it be food distribution, the economics of North/South inequities or desertification due to climate changes, they all carry the hallmark of human short-sightedness.

A basic biological need is that of healing, ensuring the maintenance of wholeness and thus survival. The environment provides for this as well as food for nutrition. The biosphere was not waiting for the evolution of multinational drug companies before there could be healthy animals! Healing is a Gaian quality as it is a very personal expression of balance and wholeness.

The relationship between healing plants and people can be seen as Gaia in action. It does not matter whether your interest is in the chemistry of secondary plant products, interactions between saponins and the human immune system, whole plant actions or the energy fields of plants, the context is one of ecological embrace.

Rediscovery of the profound relationship that exists between plants and humanity renews the old rapport in a new context, offering a way to resolve many apparently insoluble human problems. As an expression of very real and practical links with Gaia, there is an activation of ecological cycles for healing, so facilitating the work of Christ. A unique opportunity is created by the simple act of taking herbal medicines; in fact the door is opened to the possibility of a miracle of healing way beyond the removal of disease. This profound and deeply transforming miracle is facilitated by a direct experience of ecological flow and integration: an experience of belonging in the deepest sense, knowing that one is home, healed and whole. Such healing goes beyond the treatment of pathologies and the alleviation of bodily suffering that herbal remedies do so well. Rather, it is in the realm of the transcendental, the ineffable transformation that comes about through the touch of God.

It has little to do with specific herbs or health-care pro-grammes. It results from a bridging of the alienation deep within the psyche, the separation from the embrace of both nature and soul that plagues humanity. The medieval herbalist and mystic Hildegard Von Bingen talks of *viriditas*, the Green-ing power. The healing offered so abundantly and freely by the plant kingdom is indeed a greening of the human condi-tion, pointing to the reality of a new springtime. Humanity is awakening and finally becoming present within the biosphere.

In the New Testament, Jesus says, 'When two or more come together in my name, there so am I.' The Bible does not specify that they be two or more *people*, and indeed, as Christ's love embraces all beings on all planes of existence, it surely encompasses herbs. In the Christian tradition, healing is deeply aligned with the Christ and in fact is an expression of the presence of Christ. Involvement in any aspect of healing work is, similarly, an involvement in Christ's work among humanity. Could it not be said that by using herbs in healing a human being comes together with the plant in Christ's name? The words might be different, but the process and intention are fundamentally the same, only the degree of awareness of it varies.

Herbalism abounds with opportunities to experience the reality of the healing presence of nature, whether in treating disease or in hugging a tree. Approaching herbalism from its array of diverse and divergent components illuminates a field of human endeavour that is a wonderful weaving of the miraculous and the mundane. It is a therapy that encompasses anthraquinone laxatives, the spiritual ecstasy of the Amazo-nian shaman and the beauty of the flower. The limits to what might be called the path of the herbalist are only those imposed by parochial vision and constipated imagination!

4

It has been said that without vision the people die. Without a personal vision, life becomes a slow process of degeneration and decay, and without some social vision civilisation rapidly disintegrates. Such life-affirming vision is different to taking on a dogmatic belief system. It is an expression of meaning in an individual's life and must come from his or her core. A green vision of humanity's place within the family of Gaia is rapidly illuminating our culture. Herbalism, with its reverence for life and bridging between plants and people, is at the heart of this transformation.

WHAT ARE HERBS AND WHAT IS HERBALISM?

Herbs are different things to different people, with definitions varying according to area of interest and personal bias. What then is herbalism? Just saying that it is the study of herbs begs the question. The lack of clarity reflects the changing fortunes of herbalism in English-speaking cultures over the centuries. At one time herbalism was an honourable profession that laid foundations for modern medicine, botany, pharmacy, perfumery and chemistry, but as these developed and our culture's infatuation with technology and reductionism took over, herbalism was relegated to the history books or pleasantly quaint country crafts. This left a word with a variety of uses but without a cultural core. As herbalism develops afresh in what has been called the 'Herbal Renaissance', it is time for this little word to be reclaimed.

From a holistic perspective, a herb is a plant in relationship with humanity, and herbalism becomes the exploration of humanity's relationship with the plant kingdom. The dictionaries, usually the authoritative source of the 'true' meaning of words, would disagree.

The Complete Oxford Dictionary contains over three pages of definitions of words around herb and herbalist, demonstrating the importance of this field to our culture. The primary definition of *herb* reads 'A plant of which the stem does not become woody or persistent (as in a shrub or tree), but remains more or less soft and succulent, and dies down to the ground (or entirely) after flowering.' The second definition says that the term *herb* is 'applied to plants of which the leaves or stem and leaves are used for food or medicine, or in some way for their scent or flavour'. Herbalism as a subject was once the description for what is now called botany, again pointing to an important role for herbalism in the past. *The Collins English Dictionary* defines a herbalist as a person who grows, sells, collects or specialises in the use of herbs, especially medicinal herbs. It used to be the term for a descriptive botanist, although now they would probably be offended!

Botany views herbs as non-woody plants, that is they do not contain woody lignin fibres. *Dorland's Medical Dictionary* similarly defines a herb as 'a plant whose stems are soft and perishable, and which are supported chiefly by turgor pressure.' The science of ecology, the study of the inter-relationships between plants, animals and the environment, has a very specific use of the word herb. In descriptions of complex communities, such as forest, herbs are plants that are less than 12 inches high that live their life-cycles in the 'herb layer'. This would suggest that trees and shrubs such as Sarsaparilla and Cramp Bark are not herbs.

The culinary arts have explored the use of plants in many delicious ways, but usually restrict what is called a herb to those plants that smell and taste wonderful. These are usually plants rich in pleasantly aromatic volatile oils such as Basil, Peppermint or Oregano. No self-respecting chef would think of creating culinary delights with Stinking Iris (*Iris foetidimus*), Skunk Cabbage (*Symplocarpus foetida*) or Golden Seal (*Hydrastis canadensis*)! This does not mean they are not herbs, simply that they don't taste good.

In the various branches of medicine, the word usually im-plies plants that are sources for healing remedies, either in their 'crude' form or as sources of physiologically active chemicals. This can lead towards only physiologically potent plants being recognised as herbs, ignoring the gentle tonic remedies. From the perspective of the medical herbalist, a herb is any plant material that may be used in the field of health and wholeness. This may be a herb in the strictly botanical sense with a remedy such as White Horehound (*Marrubium vulgare*), or a part of a plant as in the flowers of Marigold (*Calendula officinalis*), the heart wood of the Lignum Vitae tree (*Guaiacum officinale*), the seeds of Chasteberry (*Vitex agnus-castus*) or the roots of Cone Flower (*Echinacea angustifolia*).

One general definition often given states that 'a herb is any useful plant'. However, from the perspectives of the environmentalist, it is possible to ask what plant is not useful. Indeed it could be argued that Poison Oak, Poison Ivy, Nettles and Brambles are exceptionally useful as they keep humans off that piece of land! The wholeness of the environment is vital for individual human health, implying that all plants in our environment have a medicinal role to play in planetary terms.

If the holistic context is taken in its broadest sense, then a herb is a plant in relationship with humanity, and herbalism becomes the study and exploration of the interaction between humanity and the plant kingdom. Such a stance highlights the range and depth of human dependence on plants. This relationship is at the core of agriculture, forestry, carpentry, construction, clothing, medicine and so on. In fact as coal is geologically processed wood, this broad view would include the petrochemical industry as a subset of modern herbalism!

The depth of this relationship goes way beyond such social and economic issues to the very life-sustaining mechanisms of planetary ecology. The health and well-being of the biosphere is governed by the green mantle of the Earth. Humanity's rapacious exploitation and destruction of the forests and seas strike at the very core of Gaia's life-support mechanisms. It is becoming evident that to survive the crisis at hand, humanity must learn some environmental humility and co-operate with nature. Herbalism is a unique and important expression of this co-operation within Gaia. The green world is actively healing the human world; as our birthright we are in the caring embrace of Mother Earth. It does not need to be created, simply experienced.

HERBS AND HOLISM, PARADIGM SHIFT

Medical herbalism is thriving today, using whole plants to treat whole people, facilitating the healing process within the framework of holistic medicine. It is both an art and science, and with its roots in the venerable past, it is relevant and meaningful in the present and points not only towards an exciting future for the whole of medicine but even for directions in which our society might decide to go.

It has a breadth of use as wide as any form of medicine, as herbs may be used for any condition that is medically treatable. This is not to claim that herbalism is a panacea for the ills of humanity. The ecological integration of plant activity with human physiology offers the potential for facilitating the healing process at any time in any situation. The hows and whys of this are developed throughout the book, but medical herbalism is re-asserting its relevance today as society learns about wholeness (or the lack of it).

A new understanding of health is appearing. Such a change is both in attitude and approach, and is often referred to as holistic medicine. This is a small part of a massive shift in the way we see ourselves and the issues that affect us. This has been called a paradigm shift; a change in the patterns of belief and perception that our culture has about itself. Such a shift has happened many times before. From the vantage point of history the transformation of society from the medieval world view to what we now call the Renaissance is strikingly clear. However, to the people of the time the process of change would either have been imperceptible or totally confusing, unless you were a Leonardo Da Vinci.

This development of new patterns of expectation and explanation is, of course, affecting the field of medicine. Questions are being raised about every aspect of medicine, from the nature of health and disease, to appropriate therapeutic techniques. All of which is the exploration of the new paradigm.

What then is health from the context of this new paradigm? The World Health Organisation has the clearest definition, its simplicity highlighting its profound relevance:

Health is more than simply the absence of illness. It is the active state of physical, emotional, mental and social well-being.

This is a wonderfully precise encapsulation of the perspectives of holistic medicine. This approach to medicine starts from the assumption that health is a positive and active state, that it is an inherent characteristic of whole and integrated human beings. From a holistic standpoint, a person is not a patient with a disease syndrome but a whole being. This wholeness necessitates the therapist's appreciating the mental, emotional, spiritual, social and environmental aspects of their patients' lives, as well as the physical. A holistic practitioner, of whatever specific therapy, has a deep respect for the individual's inherent capacity for self-healing. This enables a relationship of active partnership in the healing process, rather than that of an expert and a passive recipient.

Relating to the whole person is, of course, not new. It is an inherent part of the healer's heritage. From the teachings of Hippocrates onwards there has been the deeply caring support of the patient that every doctor, every herbalist, every nurse, is guided towards by their teachers. Naming and emphasising holistic medicine today is an attempt to correct the tendency in modern medicine to equate health care with the treatment of a 'disease entity'.

Holism does not pre-define any medical technique or theory. Rather it is a context in which the whole person is considered, their physical health as well as mental/emotional state, their relationships and life in the world. A medical doctor can be holistic, as can a medical herbalist or osteopath. A framework becomes apparent that can embrace a whole range of therapeutic modalities, whether labelled 'orthodox' or 'alternative'. They may all be used in a relevant and coherent way while treating the whole of a person, not simply symptoms or even a syndrome. As holistic medicine rapidly develops it is worth articulating some provisional ideas, bearing in mind that this is a time of flux.

Holistic medicine emphasises the uniqueness of the individual coming for care, for while physical, emotional, mental and spiritual aspects are acknowledged, the importance of tailoring treatment to meet the individual's broad needs is fundamental. The need to understand and treat people in the context of their family, their community and their culture is paramount.

As holistic medicine sees health as a positive state of well-being, and not simply the absence of disease, it emphasises the promotion of health and the prevention of disease. Therapeutic modalities are employed that mobilise the individual's innate capacity for self-healing. Individuals' role in their own healing process is emphasised, with much responsibility being handed back to them. While not denying the occasional necessity for swift and authoritative medical or surgical intervention, the emphasis is on helping people understand and help themselves, focusing on education and self-care rather than just treatment and the resulting dependency.

A unique and important characteristic of any holistic approach is viewing illness as an opportunity for self-discovery, not just as a misfortune. This leads to many important implications for the caring professions, perhaps best exemplified by the hospice movement. There is an appreciation of the quality of life in each of its stages and a commitment to improving it, as well as the knowledge of the illnesses that are common to it. The therapeutic importance of the setting within which health care takes place is also fundamental to holistic practice. Part of the problem with medical care is the alienation and dehumanising that tends to accompany institutions and laboratories. When the healing process is separated too far from the humanity of the people involved, there is nothing other than chemistry and surgery. The hearts of doctor and patient must meet as well as their skill and symptoms.

For a holistic practitioner there is a recognition of the social and economic conditions that perpetuate ill health, A commitment to change these factors is as much part of holistic medicine as is the emphasis on individual responsibility.

Taking all this together clearly shows why holistic medicine transforms its practitioners as well as its patients. Herbal medicine fits well into this emerging holistic paradigm. It is a healing technique that is inherently in tune with Nature, and has been described as ecological healing because of its basis in the shared ecological and evolutionary heritage with the plant kingdom through which herbal remedies work.

THERAPEUTIC ECOLOGY

Holistic medicine highlights the very personal nature of the healing process. A common idea among all holistically orientated therapists is that a human being is a self-healing individual, and at best all a medical practitioner can do is facilitate this profound inner process. Addressing pathology is relatively straightforward, but, as the WHO definition highlights, health is much more than the absence of disease, it is an active state of well-being. Self-healing is a natural birthright, as at the core of what it means to be human is a spark of the divine that moves us towards wholeness and fulfilment. It does not negate the importance of medicine and the healing arts, but provides a broad context within which to view them.

Such a self-healing individual is enmeshed in a therapeutic ecology. It is called an ecology because the various components are in relationship with each other and the wider world. The individual is seen as the core of this therapeutic ecology, embraced by four groups or branches of therapies. In the model shown in Figure 1 they are called medicine, body work, psychological and spiritual techniques. As all healing work happens within a wider picture, the pattern of relationships is itself embraced by the support of Gaia and illuminated by the miracle of Grace.

Medicine is used here to mean anything which is taken for healing purposes. Such approaches include medical herbalism, homeopathy, naturopathy and drug-based allopathic medicine. All have in common the use of some 'form' level medicine that is taken into the body to achieve the therapeutic goal. The specifics vary, of course, but all such medicines can be seen as fruits of the Earth. Whether they are in the form of a herb or synthesised drug, they share a common origin in the physical world.

Body work includes all approaches that do something with or to the physical body. Structural factors are focused on as either causation or contribution to illness. This includes the manipulative therapies such as osteopathy, chiropractic and

11

the varieties of massage, as well as surgery. Personal lifestyle will contribute exercise, dance or any expression of bodily vitality.

Work with the psyche embraces a whole array of psychological techniques, so important for identifying and treating emotional and mental factors in health and disease. All the branches of psychotherapy are involved here, but especially the more holistically orientated approaches of humanistic and transpersonal psychology. A conscious and free-flowing emotional life is fundamental to achieving any inner harmony. This does not mean that everyone must get involved in depth psychology, but that attention be given in the appropriate form for the individual's emotional needs. Mental factors are crucial as we are what we think.

Spiritual factors in human healing are becoming increasingly recognised by materialistic Western medicine. There are meditative and prayer-based techniques where the person aligns their being with the higher spirit, or those where a practitioner works with the energy body of a patient. Some openness to spirituality is vital, and it might take the form of being uplifted by a sunset, being touched by poetry or art, belief in a religion, or simply a dogma-free joy in being alive.

Holism tells us to focus on an individual's unique situation and not simply treat a diagnosed disease syndrome. In the context of this therapeutic ecology, it may be that one person diagnosed with colitis might recuperate best when treated with dietary advice, herbs and osteopathic manipulation while for another it could be drugs, psychoanalysis and surgery. Practitioners will have their firmly held opinions of the pros and cons concerning one approach or another, but the patient is always more important than his or her doctor's belief system.

Such therapeutic relationships point to the possibilities of mutual support. This may take the form of compensating for any weaknesses inherent within a particular therapy, for example homoeopathic remedies will not put a fractured arm into a splint. From a more positive perspective, co-operation can lead to synergistic support, with the whole of any treatment programme being more than the sum of its parts. A geodesic relationship develops where extraordinary potential and strength can flow from co-operation between the therapies. Differences can now lead to a celebration of the richness of therapeutic diversity and no longer be a cause for acrimonious debate and conflict.

A key insight for the practitioner is knowing the limits of both their therapy and themselves. Within the framework of this therapeutic ecology, a more appropriate avenue can be identified to direct the patient towards their healing. It should be a given that a well-qualified practitioner is skilled in their chosen healing art, but a true holistic healer will be thinking beyond their training and focusing on the needs of the sick person. This, however, raises questions about educational standards which cannot be meaningfully explored here. Suffice it to say that an MD who attends a short training in acupuncture is no more an acupuncturist than a chiropractor who does a workshop on herbs becomes a medical herbalist.

IS IT COMPLEMENTARY, ALTERNATIVE OR ORTHODOX?

This array of therapies simply comprises different modalities within the broad church of medicine. With the rapidly changing situation among the healing professions, it would be a mistake to talk of medical herbalism as a form of alternative medicine. Is it an alternative to acupuncture, osteopathy or psychiatry? Of course not: they complement each other, creating a complex of relationships where the whole is much more than the sum of the parts. In light of the unique strengths and weaknesses each approach offers, mutual support and co-operation is the way forward towards a truly holistic health service. All medical modalities are complementary within the perspective of the patient's needs.

Language often blocks communication and shared endeavour in medicine. Apparent vocabulary and jargon disparities may mask fundamental agreements of ideas and approach. On the other hand, lack of clarity obscures important differences in both guiding principles and techniques. There is an all-too-common dogmatic attachment to words and specific formulations of belief, opinion and theory. If the 'correct' words or phrases are not used then the speaker must be wrong!

Entrenched confrontation between dedicated allopathic practitioners and dedicated holistic practitioners becomes irrelevant when seen in the context of therapeutic ecology. Open-mindedness and tolerance should be characteristics common to all involved in health care, whether as practitioners, researchers, or patients. Medical modalities that have their foundations outside the biomedical model should not be ignored or discounted simply because they exemplify a different belief system. They should be respected as an enrichment of possibilities and not a challenge to the status quo.

Everyone involved in health-care provision will benefit in such a mutually supportive environment, as such cooperative endeavours bear many kinds of fruit. Health-service administrators will appreciate the economic savings gleaned from a lessening of dependence upon costly medical technology. A proportion of procedures and treatments that currently utilise expensive drugs or surgery will be undertaken by more appropriate techniques from another healing modality. For example, most run-of-the-mill gall-bladder removals could be avoided by using herbs or homoeopathic remedies, and some expensive orthopaedic techniques could be replaced with skilled osteopathy.

What then is the contribution of medical herbalism to this healing framework? That is what the rest of this book explores!

An enduring strength of herbalism is its strong foundations in traditional healing, while being at the same time part of modern science and medicine. Paradoxically, herbalism is both a wonderfully simple and staggeringly complex therapy. Its simplicity is reflected in the ease of picking Cleavers from the hedgerow or chewing on a stem of Chickweed, while its complexity is seen when trying to grasp processes that underly the multitude of biochemical interactions between all of the plant's chemical constituents and the metabolic basis of human physiology. The degree and depth of interaction are breathtaking.

Practitioners of medical herbalism have the unique possibility of their patients being introduced to their medicine! A bridge can be built between person and herb, empowering them to be present and responsible in the healing process. They can be given a packet of herb seeds, encouraging a direct experience of the life of the plant. This experience of herbal 'vitality' will be translated into a deeper rapport with the impersonal 'medicine' they take. The patient will not only get the medical benefit from the herb but also the enlivening experience of growing and preparing their own healing. If there is no garden, part of the treatment might involve a window box!

Medical herbalism will take its place at the heart of a future national holistic health service. It is not only an effective medical system, it holds out the hope of great rewards for society if embraced as a modality within an array of health-care services.

THE HISTORY OF HERBALISM

Herbalism is an ancient and venerable art that has thrived in all cultures of the world and in all historical periods until the very recent past in the industrialised West. As a constant and vital thread in human life, it is alive and well, and even in the Western world there is a rediscovery of the value of herbal medicine. The rich and colourful history of herbalism is the history of humanity itself. As a branch of medicine it has occasionally found itself on the wrong side of the establishment, but this ebb and flow of 'acceptance' is symptomatic of the changing fashions and opinions of medical and legal elites.

Apart from being very enjoyable, a brief skimming of herbalism's fascinating history reveals very little. No attempt will be made to cover it here as others have already done it extremely well. The interested reader should consult the excellent *Green Pharmacy* by Barbara Griggs, the best and most comprehensive history of herbalism yet written.

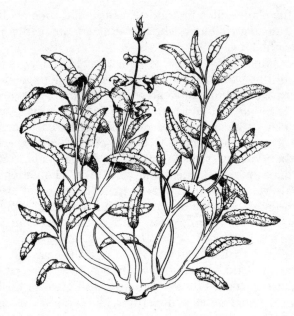

Figure 1   *Sage*

HERBALISM AND HOMOEOPATHY

As a number of therapies use plants in their healing work, confusion exists as to their differences. There are the culturally diverse medical systems of the world that use plants as the core of treatments, such as Ayurveda from India, traditional Chinese medicine and Islamic Unani medicine. Among Western therapies homoeopathy, aromatherapy and the Bach flower remedies make extensive use of herbs. The majority of drugs used in orthodox medicine are either derived from plants or are actually plant products.

Homoeopathy is the main system of medicine other than medical herbalism that utilises plants in the treatment of disease, though in a fundamentally different way to medical herbalism. There is a common misconception that these two healing modalities are the same because they both employ plants. Indeed, herbs are used by both approaches but in radically different ways, reflecting differences of philosophy and therapeutics. The holistic perspective being explored by their practitioners can complement each other, but only when the strengths and weaknesses of each are acknowledged and understood.

As with other approaches to holistic medicine, homoeopathy looks at the patient's total picture, both body and mind, within the social setting of their lives. The system originated in Germany around 1800, with the work of Samuel Hahnemann. He treated disease with a very low dose of drugs which themselves produced similar symptoms to those of the disease itself. This is the basis of the principle that 'like treats like'.

About 60 per cent of homoeopathic remedies are botanical in nature, the rest being minerals, animal products or 'nosodes'. These last remedies are highly diluted extracts of diseased tissue. These medicines are administered in extremely diluted form and are thought to work by influencing the vital force within the human body. The more the dose of the remedy is reduced, the more its potency is enhanced. This is why the homoeopathic process of dilution is known as 'potentiation'. The dilution of one part of the active remedy in ten parts of the solvent (usually water) is known as a potency of 1X. A one in a hundred dilution is 2X and so on to 200X dilution. A homoeopathic mother tincture is similar to an ordinary herbal tincture.

A problem that gets in the way of mutual understanding between the two therapies is the application of the concept of like treating like. Many of the herbs in the homoeopathic Materia Medica are prescribed in dilution to treat symptom pictures that a full dose of the herb supposedly causes. This may be the case with very strong or poisonous herbs such as Belladona or Gelsemium, but the medical herbalist has problems with the homoeopath's ideas about many of the remedies both systems share. An example is the homoeopathic remedy pulsatilla, known as Pasque Flower (*Anemome pulsatilla*) to the herbalist. A comparison of the symptom picture given for the homoeopathic remedy is very similar to the indications for herbal dosages of the plant. As both approaches use the herb to treat similar things, this would appear to contradict the core idea.

The value of homoeopathy in health care is undeniable, but its use of plants is in no way 'herbal'. Selecting either therapy should be based upon attraction to one or other of their philosophical contexts recognising that there is little or no sharing of botanical medicine.

THE INTERNATIONAL CONTEXT OF HERBAL MEDICINE

Herbalism is a common bond between the peoples and cultures of the world. This shared experience of alleviating humanities suffering through plant medicines bridges cultural divides, religous differences and racial conflicts. The worldwide knowledge and wisdom that the herbalist offers is a unique and invaluable resource that cannot be regained once lost. The important and valiant efforts of ethnopharmacologists and others to find healing plants so that patentable drugs may be developed miss the central insight of humanity use of herbs. There is a relationship between a culture and its plant environment within which the herbalist plays a pivotal role. Herbalism is more than knowledge about healing plants; it is the experience and wisdom that comes from the relationship between humanity and plants.

The World Health Organisation (WHO) has recognised this important insight and is now promoting the development of what it calls traditional medicine. At the 30th World Health Assembly in 1977 the World Health Organisation adopted a resolution urging interested governments to give:

> adequate importance to the utilisation of their traditional systems of medicine, with appropriate regulations as suited for their national health systems.[2]

This led to a worldwide effort by the WHO to enhance traditional medicine in its various forms. 'Traditional medicine' is taken as implying all the knowledge and practices used in the prevention, diagnosis and elimination of physical, mental or social imbalance. These are based on experience and observation handed down from generation to generation, whether by word of mouth or written down. It includes highly developed systems such as Ayurveda from India and the complexities of traditional Chinese medicine, as well as collections of simple local home remedies.

Traditional medicine, of which herbalism is the most important form, fits perfectly into the World Health Organisation's holistic definition of health (see p.8). From this perspective the possibility opens for dialogue and integration between current scientific approaches to health and the older traditional techniques. The assembly affirmed that all medicine is modern in so far as it is directed towards the goal of providing health care. The essential difference between various systems of medicine is that of their cultural context rather than goals or effects.

As an international body, there is a fundamental recognition on the part of the WHO that all traditions have value, and that any world view as seen from the belief system of any one particular tradition is inherently limited. Thus from the cloisters of a Western medical school the view of reality is as limited and limiting as that from a shaman's hut in West Africa. All perspectives have value in any worldwide approach to health for all.

The fundamentally holistic approach of much traditional medicine views the person as a whole being living within a broad ecological spectrum of factors affecting health. There is a widely held belief across many different approaches to traditional medicines that disease is brought about by an imbalance of the person in their total ecological system and not simply by a single cause or pathogen.

The WHO has identified a number of intrinsic qualities that justify promoting traditional medicine, the most noteworthy of which are:

- Traditional medicine has intrinsic value and in recognition of this it should be promoted and its potential developed for the wider use and benefit of mankind.
- Traditional medicine is already the people's own health-care system and is well accepted by them.
- Traditional medicine has certain advantages over imported systems of medicine because as an integral part of the people's culture, it is particularly effective in solving certain cultural health problems.

- Traditional medicine contributes greatly to scientific medicine, thus justifying its development from the Western biomedical perspective.

These are some of the reasons why the WHO considers it so vital to promote and develop traditional medicine. In practical terms perhaps the best reason for the rapid advance of their programme is that it is one of the ways to achieve the aim of total health care by the year 2000, as the burgeoning human population of the world would be covered using acceptable, safe and economically feasible methods. An exciting development that promises many practical insights for the 'developed' West, is the move to integrate traditional methods of healing with 'Western' medicine. Acknowledging the value of herbs and the healing perspective in which they are used, many countries in the world are co-operating with the WHO in programmes that integrate traditional approaches with the scientific techniques of modern medicine. This synthesis is a goal that will be achieved in the foreseeable future. A WHO report proposes some interesting prerequisites for integration, including:

- Provision of valid factual data to overcome the current lack of information. This may then be used to help convince decision-makers, professional health personnel and the population at large of the value of integration.
- Legal recognition of the therapies and therapists to ensure socio-political acceptability and access to resources.
- The early establishment of dialogue among practitioners of differing systems. This should eliminate prejudice and hopefully develop more acceptable attitudes.

A move towards some form of integration is inevitable in Britain and the rest of the Western world as the limits of the value of allopathic medicine are reached. A well-integrated holistic health service would offer the benefits of all approaches to health care, not simply one system or another. We should be holistic in our national services as well as the treatment of the individual.

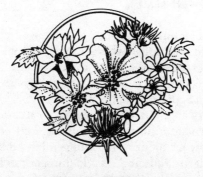

2 · DO HERBS WORK?

Why is this question asked at all? In most of the world it would simply not be posed, for why question the obvious? We in the technological West, however, have built our whole culture upon questioning the obvious!

While the question might imply fundamental doubts about the validity of medical herbalism as a therapeutic technique, it also demonstrates a profound ignorance of the daily reality of the herbal practitioner. The medical herbalists of the world have abundant evidence that their remedies work, as does the parent using gripe water for a baby with colic. There is also a wealth of evidence from the professional journals of medicine and science. Anyone who considers herbalism quackery or herbs at best placebo medicine is simply demonstrating their ignorance.

In the next few pages evidence will be presented that shows that plants can play an important part in health care, but this does not mean that herbs are always the therapy of choice. Herbalism is not the best technique when troubled with a broken arm, or for the very acute life-threatening infections such as meningitis. The diversity of health-care techniques available is something to celebrate, not a cause for conflict and exclusivity. All can work together and support each other. One technique's strength can support the weaknesses of another. Allopathic, herbal and homoeopathic medicine are examples where much mutual benefit flows when co-operation rather than dogmatic conflict is the key-note. The needs of the patient are always more important than the beliefs of the practitioner.

Health care is almost exclusively an expression of technology in Western culture. This is all well and good as far as it goes, but problems arise where such an approach does not go. Modern medicine, in placing so much value in the analytical, reductionist techniques of science, has lost sight of the Hippocratic vision of wholeness. The perceptual tools of biomedical science blind it to the possibilities and even the existence of the state of health that is brought about through a movement towards human wholeness. Providing a therapeutic rationale for medical herbalism is, however, an important and necessary step. This does not limit or deny the value of other approaches or even pre-define how to use the plant remedies, it simply provides one path in the exploration of this vast field of knowledge, a field that offers so much in exciting therapeutic possibilities.

Herbs can play a unique role in all healing work, as any health problem that is medically treatable will benefit from herbal therapy. As a therapy medical herbalism is especially indicated in chronic, or long-standing problems. For most common acute medical problems it will also be useful, but occasionally the herbs may not act fast enough or be sufficiently specific in their mode of action. This is especially the case with life-threatening infections. With degenerative diseases of all kinds reaching epidemic proportions throughout the Western world, herbal therapeutics may now be coming into its own. Diseases that reflect a degenerative breakdown within the body respond notoriously badly to orthodox treatments, but will often do well with appropriate herbal therapy. Prevention of disease and removal of factors that might lead to illness is one of the strong points of medical herbalism. As explored elsewhere in the book, there is a well-developed approach to using herbs for prevention and the maintenance of wholeness. In fact holistic approaches to health emphasise the whole area of wellness rather than illness. Medical herbalism is most effective at supporting the body's innate integrating and self-healing processes.

Demonstrating or 'proving' that herbs work is not always a straightforward matter. The first step is to ascertain what form the 'proof' needs to be in for the person concerned. For an individual, sick or well, there need only be the subjective experience of personal benefit gained from using herbal medicine. For others it may be a similarly subjective observation of another's experience. However, for the medical establishment and many people who perceive the world from this perspective, such subjective experiences are invalid. There must be some objective, quantifiable and reproducible data. When herbs are examined in this way, it will take the form of laboratory or clinical findings which are then put through statistical analysis. Evidence and proof become a dispassionate mathematical process rather than a messy human one. The striving for scientific objectivity has obscured the reality of working with human beings with all their diversity and idiosyncrasies. A book like this one is not the place to explore the strengths and weaknesses of

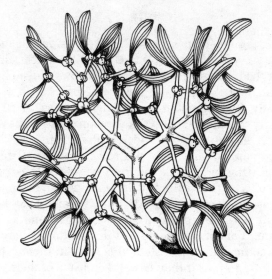

Figure 2   *Mistletoe*

the scientific method. However, some clear problems arise for the medical herbalist in a world where the arbiters of medical veracity still consider the Cartesian paradigm to be the truth, the whole truth and nothing but the truth.

On the most basic experiential levels it is easy to show that herbs 'work'. There are a range of remedies that have a demonstrable impact upon human physiology. One of the most widely used plants in the world is Senna (*Cassia* spp.), an effective laxative that works through a biochemical triggering of bowel movements. Within twelve hours of ingestion there is a triggering of muscular contractions along the colon which leads to an emptying of the bowels. This does not involve belief, placebo effect, or even knowledge that the herb has been ingested. In other words, such a dramatic experience proves that herbs work. Similarly the ubiquitous weed Dandelion has leaves which give a strong diuretic impact, equivalent to the strength of the drug frusemide. The French name of one Dandelion, *Pisse en Lit*, hints at its diuretic strength. Not a herb to drink last thing at night!

VALERIAN

As an example of a specific plant consider the relaxing nervine remedy Valerian. It is a beautiful and useful plant with a bad press! Its characteristically 'unusual' aroma unfortunately keeps many people at bay. A pity, as it is a remedy that offers much relief and ease to struggling humanity in the face of the tensions and stress of our world. It has an ancient and worldwide history. Scholars have concluded that it is the same plant that the Greek herbalist Dioscorides called Phu, because of its offensive smell. It was first called Valeriana in the ninth century and was later known as All Heal in medieval England, where it was considered a spice and perfume as well as medicine. Cats are attracted to this wonderful herb, and it can sometimes induce a state of ecstasy in them. They will roll around in it as if they have taken leave of their senses, a far more impressive display than with catnip.

A number of herbs belong to the genus *Valeriana*, but three are commonly used: *V. officinalis*, *V. sitchensis* and *V. wallichii*. It is collected in the autumn, as after a season's growth the roots will be rich in material that has been created during the growing season. A range of chemical constituents have been found, but as with all herbal remedies it is a mistake to try to understand the plant from these chemicals alone. The healing gift of Valerian is much more than simply the effects of constituents like valepotriates. The practitioner of herbal medicine can glean much of value from biochemical research that can augment clinical experience but never replace it. As with all medicinal plants, Valerian contains a complex of active constituents, making meaningful analysis extremely difficult. Even detailed and thorough investigation does not reveal a single active constituent in this well-known medicinal plant, highlighting the fact that the therapeutic effect depends on the interaction of the plant's constituents as a whole.

The peculiar bouquet of Valerian is actually produced by exposure to oxygen in the air during the drying process. Over a period of time, a number of components of the volatile oil in the roots hydrolyse to isovaleric acid. Very little is present in the fresh root, which has a pleasant aroma. The older the dried herb the stronger the smell of isovaleric acid, but not necessarily stronger in effect. This volatile oil has anti-microbial, carminative and relaxing properties. Pharmacological research has identified constituents known as valepotriates in the root. These are not present in the fresh root itself and therefore not in Valerian tincture or extracts prepared from it; they only develop on processing. A whole series of valepotriates has been isolated, and their actions have been found to be different, and in part opposite. In addition to relatively strong sedative properties they have a regulatory effect on the autonomic system. One fraction has a suppressant effect, another a stimulant one, so that in combination they have an equalising effect that has been referred to as amphoteric. Alkaloids are also present that have blood-pressure-lowering effects.

Valerian has a wide range of applications, but it is used

mainly in cases of anxiety, nervous sleeplessness, and the bodily symptoms of tension such as muscle-cramping or indigestion. It may be used safely in situations where tension and anxiety are causing problems. This may manifest in purely psychological and behavioural ways or also with body symptoms. Valerian will help in most cases. For some people it can be an effective mild pain reliever.

As one of the best gentle and harmless herbal sleeping remedies, it enhances the natural body process of slipping into sleep and making the stresses of the day recede. For people who do not need as much sleep as they once did, it also eases lying awake in bed, ensuring that it becomes a restful and relaxing experience. This is often as revivifying as sleep itself, and indeed such rest is all that is necessary in more cases than not. Yet this is far from a merely suggestive effect or placebo; a genuine pharmacodynamic action is present. It is only necessary to use the right method and, as cannot be stressed enough, to make sure that the dose is not too small.

The true nature of sleep still remains a mystery. Everybody goes through stages of REM (rapid eye movement) sleep, a stage where dreaming is associated with minor involuntary muscle jerks and rapid eye movements, indicating that active processes are occurring in the brain. It is important not to suppress this dreaming stage, for it is necessary to man and in no way disruptive. Emotional experiences are processed by the mind in those dreams, and much that is arising both from the unconscious and daily life is balanced and harmonised. This should not be interfered with, but unfortunately sleeping pills have a marked impact on REM. Herbal sleeping remedies do not interfere with this process as they are not powerful enough to suppress these necessary REM phases. Rather, they induce relaxation at night, helping body and mind to be ready for sleep.

The research into Valerian is confirming the traditional experience of the herbalist. In one study Valerian produced a significant decrease in subjectively evaluated sleep scores and an improvement in sleep quality. Improvement was most notable amongst those who considered themselves poor or irregular sleepers and smokers. Dream recall was relatively unaffected by Valerian.[3] When the effect of Valerian root on sleep was studied in healthy, young people, it reduced perceived sleep latency and the wake time after sleep onset. In other words they experienced an easier and quicker descent into sleep.[4] A combination of Valerian and Hops was given to people whose sleep was disturbed by heavy traffic noise. Taking the herbs well before retiring reduced the noise-induced disturbance of a number of sleep-stage patterns.[5]

Much research has centred on Valerian's effects upon smooth muscle, demonstrating that it is a powerful and safe muscle relaxant.[6] It can be safely used in muscle cramping, uterine cramps and intestinal colic. Its sedative and anti-spasmodic action can be partially ascribed to the valepotriates and to a lesser extent to the sesquiterpene constituents of the volatile oils.[7] Among other effects, Valerian decreases both spontaneous and caffeine-stimulated muscular activity, significantly reduces aggressiveness of animals, and decreases a number of measurable processes in the brain.[8]

Italian researchers compared the relaxing properties of Valerian and a number of other plants on the muscles of the digestive tract. Hawthorn and Valerian were the best, followed by Passion Flower and Chamomile. Especially interesting was the finding that combining all the herbs acted in a synergistic way, being relaxing at low dosage levels.[9]

Valerian is used worldwide as a relaxing remedy in hypertension and stress-related heart problems. There is an effect here beyond simple nerve relaxation, as Valerian contains alkaloids that are mild hypotensives, or blood-pressure reducers. Such use is recognised and respected by the World Health Organisation. They promote research and development of traditional medicine that recognise the importance of using whole plants and going beyond the test tube for meaningful results. In WHO-sponsored studies in Bulgaria, traditional herbs known for their healing effect in cardiovascular problems were considered. Results of clinical examination of patients using such herbs are impressive. Valerian is one such herb whose use was validated. Others are Garlic, Geranium, European Mistletoe, Olive, and Hawthorn.

It is possible to enhance different aspects of the herb's effects by combining it with other remedies. For tension and anxiety it will combine well with Skullcap, while for sleep Hops or Passion Flower would be better. In cases of nervous indigestion use it with Chamomile or Lavender and for muscular cramps with Cramp Bark. Nature has provided humanity with many plants that help relax and soothe the mind. Our forests and meadows abound with herbs that would help avoid the need for tranquillisers and sleeping pills. If we were more in tune with the natural world, the craziness that brings about the tension in our lives would be eased anyway.

Valerian is beyond doubt a good sedative, but to be effective it has to be prescribed in sufficiently high dosage. The tincture is the most widely used preparation and is always useful, provided that the single dose is not counted in drops, but that ½–1 teaspoonful is given, and indeed sometimes 2 teaspoonfuls at one time. It is almost pointless to give ten or twenty drops of Valerian tincture. Overdosage is highly unlikely, even with very much larger doses. For situations of extreme stress where a sedative or muscle-relaxant effect is needed fast, the single dose of 1 teaspoonful may be repeated two or three times at short intervals.

If Valerian tea is to be effective, at least 2 teaspoons of the dried herb are used for each cup of tea prepared. With these doses expect a good relaxing, anti-spasmodic and sleep-inducing effect, and above all rapid sedation in states of excitement. Another popular method of preparation is a cold maceration: a glass of cold water is poured over 2 teaspoonfuls of Valerian root and left to stand for 8–10 hours. A night-time dose is thus set up in the morning, and a dose for the mornings is prepared at night.

SECONDARY PLANT PRODUCTS

Consult any good herbal and you will find listed under each plant what chemical constituents have been found. This is an unfortunate example of the 'pseudo-science' that plagues herbalism when it tries to become scientifically respectable. There are many thousands of different chemical molecules present in each cell of every plant, which may be considered as a bio-evolved whole, with each individual chemical fulfilling a role within the greater whole. Constituent lists are shorthand for both the herbalist and pharmacologist to identify possible actions and uses of the plant. When this information is taken out of context of the whole it becomes almost meaningless. The rest of the chemical complex within the herb may be seen as equivalent to the complex within what we eat. The nutritional matrix of plant biochemistry profoundly modifies the activity of specific chemicals. Assimilation of an 'active ingredient', its metabolism, transportation by the blood, availability at its site of activity and many other factors are affected and modified by the whole biochemical complex in the plant.

A simple differentiation can be made between what have been called primary and secondary plant products. The primary plant products are the whole range of molecules involved in the fundamental life processes of the plant. This embraces photosynthesis, respiration, growth and repro-duction. These multitudinous chemicals have roles to play in the unfolding life of the plant, but another group appears to have no direct impact on the plant's physiology. They have been called secondary plant products because they play no primary role in the plant's life processes. It is often these very chemicals that the pharmacologists credit with medicinal value. In light of the ideas of the Gaia Hypothesis as it applies to herbalism, it could be said that plant chemistry and its relationship to humanity is Gaia in action.

These secondary plant products have been the key to the development of the overwhelming majority of chemical drugs used today. The ever-increasing volume of research published about them is a rich vein for both herbalist and doctor. The overriding proviso, however, is that the information must be tempered by knowing that it tells us little about the whole herb.

A word about the names of plant constituents. While they all have chemical descriptive nomenclature, they often have simpler names given to them by the discovering pharmacologist, usually based on the Latin botanical name. This often means that to the non-specialist they appear obtuse in the extreme. An example is the bitter sesquiterpene Cnicin. This was first found in Blessed Thistle, whose botanical name is *Cnicus benedictus*, thus explaining why it was called Cnicin. While this might seem obscure, it is preferable to the chemical nomenclature that describes it as an ester of 3,4-dihydroxy-1-butene-2 carboxylic acid with a sesquiterpene lactone!

Secondary plant products include such things as alkaloids, glycosides, xanthines and many others. A brief review of three of these groups will be illuminating.

FLAVONES AND FLAVONOIDS

An important group of plant constituents are the flavones and flavonoids. The name derives from the fact that they are often yellow in colour, from the Latin *flavus* meaning yellow. There are well over 2,000 compounds in this group, which are among the commonest and widest-spread biologically active substances found in plants. They have a great range of properties, but simply to list the physiological effects of these chemicals can obscure the fact that they work in a complex, synergistic way. The specifics described here are not separate but inter-related at the metabolic level in both plant and human, and not all of the flavones or plants containing them will have all these properties.

Pharmacology has shown these seemingly ubiquitous chemicals to have a gentle and beneficial impact on a whole range of organs and physiological processes. The heart, blood vessels, liver, immune system, connective tissue, adrenal glands, kidneys, musculature and nervous system may all benefit from herbs that contain flavones and flavonoids.

An anti-oxidant effect has been found, which helps prevent the formation of free radicals and a group of natural body chemicals called leucotrines, known to promote inflammation. Flavones also potentiate the action of vitamin C by blocking its oxidation. With the new insights about the role of free radicals in ageing, auto-immune disease and many other fundamental health issues, the anti-oxidant potential of flavone-containing herbs opens exciting therapeutic possibilities. The anti-inflammatory activity commonly found in flavone-containing herbs is possibly due to this inhibition of the formation of leucotrines.

Some flavones strengthen connective tissue through an inhibitory effect on hyaluronidase, an enzyme that breaks down connective tissue. By blocking the activity of this enzyme, the strength and integrity of connective tissue ground substance is maintained and even increased. Catechin, rutin, hesperidin and querctin are common flavones that have this property. This may be a partial explanation for the regenerative effect observed with herbal treatments on connective tissue, especially following injury.

They also stabilise capillary permeability. This property enables the tissues of the body to guard against bruising due to capillary fragility. It was the discovery of this property that led to the coining of the name vitamin P for what have been called bioflavonoids. The reduction in leakage is believed to be related to histamine metabolism. Rutin containing Buckwheat is a good example.

Some of the medical herbalist's favourite blood-pressure-lowering remedies (hypotensives) contain flavones that are markedly hypotensive. Additionally there is a unique toning of the cardiac muscle itself. This is thought to be due to the dilation of coronary arteries and thus an increase of oxygen availability to the heart muscle. Hawthorn is the best example here. A gentle sedative action combined with a relaxation of muscle spasm supports the worldwide use of flavone-rich plants, such as Linden, as relaxing remedies.

An immuno-stimulating role has been demonstrated, supporting the long-held assertion of herbalists around the world that herbs can play a fundamental role in therapeutic programmes directed at the immune system. Some of these plant biochemicals stimulate the production of antibodies, T-cells and lymphocytes. A wonderful property that appears to be new to medical science is a protective effect on liver cells in the face of chemical toxicity. This anti-hepatotoxic action is discussed in the section on *Milk Thistle* (see p. 83), a herb rich in silymarin.

In addition there is a whole plethora of other important effects that should catch the eye of any open-minded therapist. In the laboratory a weakly oestrogenic effect was found as well as effects on corticosteroid metabolism. Diuretic herbs often contain flavones that supply this action. Anti-microbial flavones have also been found. Some of these plant constituents lower elevated blood-sugar levels. Last, but not least, an anti-neoplastic effect has been demonstrated.

Table 1   Examples of herbs containing flavones and flavonoids

Herbs	Primary flavone/flavonoid
Arnica (*Arnica montana*)	Quercetin, kaemferol
Roman Chamomile (*Anthemus nobile*)	Apigenin, essential oil
Marigold (*Calendula officinalis*)	Isorhamnetin, quercetin
Hawthorn (*Crataegus spp.*)	Quercetin, apigenin, hyperoside, rutin
German Chamomile (*Matricaria recutita*)	0.5–3% of total are flavonoids
Cowslip (*Primula veris*)	Quercetin, gossypetin
Elder (*Sambucus nigra*)	Quercetin, rutin, hyperoside
Meadowsweet (*Filipendula ulmaria*)	Spiraeoside, hyperoside, avicularin
Linden Flowers (*Tilia coradata*)	Quercetin, kaempferol, myricetin
Mullein (*Verbascum thapsis*)	2–4% of total are flavonoids
Horsetail (*Equisetum arvense*)	Luteolin, isoquercetin, equisetrin
Motherwort (*Leonurus cardiaca*)	Rutin
Golden Rod (*Solidago virgaurea*)	Rutin, quecitrin, isoquercitrin, astragalir
Milk Thistle (*Silybum marianum*)	Silybin, silymarin

SAPONINS

Another important group of plant constituents are the saponins, found in over 500 genera of plants. They have been shown to have many valuable therapeutic properties, but always remember that the specifics detailed below are not separate but inter-related at the metabolic level in both the plant and person. Repeatedly it is found that the effects of the whole plant in people are not reproducible by simply giving 'active ingredients'.

Research on plant saponins is starting to lay the foundations for an understanding of the important but vague herbal concepts of tonics, alteratives and adaptogens. Western medicine has neglected such ideas as having no basis in fact. This is not so; rather it was a reflection of research procedures that could not recognise such complex and multifactorial processes. In studying saponins, insights into the process of 'toning' are being gained. A unique immuno-modulating effect has been found that promises much in these times of immune-system disease reaching epidemic proportions. Saponins appear to have a profound, yet little understood, stimulating effect upon the reticulo-endothelial system and the white cell macrophages of the mononuclear phagocyte system (MPS). In biochemical terms it is the MPS that removes much waste matter from the blood – in other words it 'cleanses' the blood. This sounds a lot like the alterative action described elsewhere in the book.

A protective effect upon liver cells in the face of toxic poisoning or degenerative disease is probably mediated through impact upon the liver's immune-system cells, the Kupffer cells. Saponin-containing herbs have also been shown to stimulate the production of interferon in the body. The adaptogenic action of herbs such as Ginseng and Siberian Ginseng is thought to be largely due to saponins. Hormonal modulation is found with a number of herbs impacting blood levels of various hormones.

As with flavones, there are a range of other specific effects found with different saponins. A well-documented but little understood effect is the lowering of blood-cholesterol levels. Anti-microbial, expectorant, anti-inflammatory, anti-catarrhal and diuretic actions in a plant are often contributed to by the presence of saponins.

Table 2   Examples of herbs that contain saponins

Herbs	Common name
Achillea millefolium	Yarrow
Arctium lappa	Burdock
Astragalus membranaceus	Astragalus
Calendula officinalis	Marigold
Caulophyllum thalictroides	Blue Cohosh
Chionanthus virginicus	Fringetree
Digitalis purpurea	Foxglove
Dioscorea spp.	Wild Yam
Eleutherococcus senticosus	Siberian Ginseng
Gentiana lutea	Gentian
Glycyrrhiza spp.	Liquorice
Panax ginseng	Korean Ginseng
Panax quinquifolius	American Ginseng
Phytolacca americana	Poke
Rumex crispus	Yellow Dock
Salvia officinalis	Sage
Smilax spp.	Sarsaparilla
Symphytum officinale	Comfrey
Taraxacum officinale	Dandelion
Verbascum thapsis	Mullein

AROMA AND TERPENES

Volatile oils are another group of plant constituents attracting increasing attention from both researchers and therapists. The beautiful fragrances of flowers, the wonderful essences used in aromatherapy, could be described in the reductionist language of biochemistry as monoterpene complexes. However, it would be better to see this the other way around. The aridity of chemistry is uplifted and illuminated by the reality of flower fragrance. The ineffable, indescribable wonder of a flower's unique fragrance is not reduced by knowledge of the chemistry involved, rather it brings the aroma through in the realm of mental understanding.

These are chemically complex molecules classified on the number of basic terpene units present. Plants have the ability to produce almost an endless number of chemical variations on a single chemical structure, the simple isoprenoid unit with five carbon atoms. Thus we find monoterpenes, diterpenes, sesquiterpenes, etc. There were estimated to be over 1,200 sesquiterpenes, alone known of in 1976. The number of terpenoids produced by plants is larger than that of any group of natural substances, including essential oils and resins, steroids, carotenoids, and rubber. Members of this group can be found to represent all the important pharmacological properties needed in medicine, from anaesthetics and anti-inflammatories to hypotensives and vitamins. A brief look at the range of properties shown by the volatile oil monoterpenes will demonstrate the importance of these plant constituents.

At one time various essential oils and their component terpenes were used in orthodox medicine for combating infections, particularly those of the bronchial and urinary tracts, and in preventing infection of burns and wounds. Since the advent of the sulphonamides and the antibiotics, they are seldom used by allopaths today. However the monoterpenes still find extensive application as disinfectants. Because phenol was often used for the comparison of the efficacy, the 'carbolic acid coefficient' shows how much a compound is more efficacious than phenol, and the antiseptic activity of these oils is often far in excess of the chemical. These oils are among the best known of herbal medicines with their antiseptic and disinfectant properties. Thyme oil, rich in the monoterpene thymol, is 20 times more antiseptic than phenol. Thymol and carvacrol are still used extensively in mouthwashes, and various monoterpenes are incorporated in toothpastes, in which their mild antiseptic properties, coupled with their stimulation of blood circulation in the gums, are beneficial.

They are important in the treatment and prevention of diseases caused by fungi, insects and intestinal worms. For example, thymol inhibits not only bacterial growth but also the growth of yeast and moulds. It is used in laboratories for the preservation of urine and other easily perishable specimens. Ascaridole is the chief constituent of Chenopodium oil or American Wormseed oil, which until quite recently was an official anthelmintic. It is effective against several types of parasitic intestinal worms in humans, especially against roundworms, but also against hookworms. The high toxicity of ascaridole to the host led to considerable opposition to its continued clinical use. Chenopodium oil and ascaridole are thus seldom used in human medicine. They are more often applied in veterinary medicine against certain liver flukes.

Several essential oils possess insect-repellent properties. The best-known example is citronellal. On the other hand, a number of monoterpenes exhibit a pronounced attraction for certain insects, and it is probable that the combination of attractant and repellent properties of essential oils plays a role of considerable importance in the vegetable kingdom, just as their mild antibacterial and antifungal properties serve to protect the plant against noxious bacteria and fungi.

Many of the simpler terpenes are characterised by the possession of irritant properties. Certain essential oils are used externally as counter-irritant in the form of embrocations and liniments. They produce an initial feeling of warmth and smarting, which is often followed by a mild local anaesthesia, making them valuable in anti-pruritic preparations. Similar preparations are used to relieve rheumatic pain and neuralgia and in the treatment of the common cold and bronchitis.

This mild irritant action helps explain the expectorant and diuretic effects of many herbs. Monoterpenoids containing essential oils are also used as inhalants with stimulating expectorant properties due to their mild irritation of the bronchioles. Certain essential oils, such as oil of Juniper, are used as diuretics because they produce irritation in the kidneys. Buchu, a valuable herbal diuretic, contains diosphenol which has a mild irritant effect upon the nephrons of the kidney, stimulating the movement of water across the membranes and so removal of water from the body. However, this does little to explain the tonic effects of Buchu upon the whole of the urinary system.

Another important group of essential oils is the group acting on the central nervous system. They can work in a number of different ways, producing muscle relaxation, central stimulation, central sedation or narcotic effects. The best known essential oil with sedative activity is Valerian oil. Calamus oil, Melissa oil and Lavender oil also have a sedative effect.

In a study of the active constituents of Lemon Balm, the researchers concluded that a whole complex of interacting chemicals are responsible for the plant's sedative and anti-spasmodic actions. The sedative effect also occurs with small dosages. In the anti-spasmodic activity, some terpenoids of the distillate attain values that can be compared with papaverine. The total content of essential oils create additional pharmacological effects that qualitatively and quantitatively surpass the effect of particular terpenoids. *In other words the whole is more than the sum of the parts.*

An unusual structural type of monoterpenes, called iridoids, have a number of medical applications. Aucubin has an anti-microbial effect against some bacteria. The long-known herbal claims for the blood-pressure-lowering effects of Olive leaves, have been reproduced in the laboratory using an iridoid called oleuropein. Investigation of this constituent of Olive leaves showed it to be hypotensive, as well as dilating coronary arteries, normalising heart rhythms and acting as an anti-spasmodic.

Anti-inflammatory action is shown by harpagoside, first isolated from Devil's Claw (*Harpagophytum procumbens*). This provides the basis for an explanation of the observed anti-rheumatic effects of this herb discussed elsewhere in this book.

The bitter tonic herbs are often rich in iridoids. The broad tonic activity of these remedies, as well as the specific actions on the liver and gut, should provide a strong hint to the pharmacologists to study these carefully. Anti-leukemic activity has been shown in an iridoid from *Allamanda cathartica*, called allamandin. This large and important group of plant ingredients includes active anti-inflammatories, anti-spasmodics, bitters and anti-tumour agents.[10]

A remedy long used throughout Europe for wound healing and ulcer treatments is Marigold (*Calendula officinalis*). Part of its healing power appears to be based on the presence of terpenes. A triterpene glycoside called Calendulozide B exerted a marked anti-ulcerous and sedative action. In a broad-spectrum check of physiological impact it did not have any effect on the cardiovascular system, the tone of intestinal smooth muscles, kidney function or on the biligenic function of the liver. The researchers say the drug is devoid of locally irritating properties and an insignificant toxicity.[11] If this is the case with an extracted constituent, much more can be claimed for the whole plant.

HERBS, FERTILITY AND CONTRACEPTION

Great attention is being given to plants with potential anti-fertility properties. These may act through effects upon sperm motility and viability, implantation of the fertilised egg or a rejection effect within the uterus. The biochemistry of these pathways is complex, and the study of plants having such effects is revealing new mechanisms all the time.

The planetary crisis that is upon us has the population explosion as a major component, and the WHO has put great emphasis on the search for a safe, cheap and socially acceptable form of contraception. Part of this vital work has focused upon folk use of anti-fertility herbs. Very recent published work has highlighted the Mexican plants known collectively as Zoapatle.[12] All the work referred to in this section has been published since 1981. Zoapatle is a decoction made from *Montanoa tomentosa* which has been used as an oral contraceptive in traditional Mexican medicine for many centuries. Records of the use of this fascinating herb go back to Spanish reports of 1529, though, of course, its use goes back a lot further. Many historical, biological, ethnobotanical, agricultural, clinical and chemical studies have been done, mostly by Mexican scientists. It is perhaps because this excellent Mexican research was published in Spanish that it was largely ignored in Britain and America until recently.[13]

Zoapatle has been used in Mexico for the last five centuries for the induction of labour, treatment of post-partum bleeding problems, and as a menses inducer. Today, it is sold in street markets, and its long documented history of use could be taken as indirect evidence of a lack of toxicity. This assumption that the herbalist often makes has for once been confirmed by rigorous pharmacological and clinical studies. The empirical observations of the therapist and the witness of history are augmented by the toxicologists' findings that *Monantoa* is completely safe.[14]

Attempts to identify the nature of the plant's activity have shown a great variation of effects on the uterus among wild plants. This should remind us that there is great ecological variation in all plants' biological activity. Nature is diverse and variable, not a standardised factory any more than people are! Much of the research has focused upon establishing standards for optimum environmental conditions and effectiveness of different varieties. After some confusion about different species it has been established that both *Montanoa tomentosa* and *M. frutescens* should be the primary focus of research.

Its anti-fertility characteristics are the possible starting-point for development of a new oral contraceptive agent which works by stimulating an evacuation of the implanted egg in the uterus. A confusingly ambivalent uterine response was found, the plant stimulating different responses at different times. This is due to different activity depending upon the phase of the oestrous cycle or stage of pregnancy, the hallmark of a primarily normalising remedy. Its chemistry and physiological activity suggest that it does not work in the oestrogenic way that formulations such as the birth control 'pill' do. Zoapatle seems to possess a quite unique anti-fertility activity.[15]

In laboratory tests the species usually described, *Montanoa tomentosa*, did not influence sperm motility or viability, but *Montanoa frutescens* had immediate and constant inhibitory effect upon motility and decreased cell viability.[16] When used as an intrauterine administration in laboratory rats, markedly different results were obtained depending which species was used. *Montanoa frutescens* produced an almost total inhibition of implantation sites, while *Montanoa tomentosa*, prepared and administered in the same fashion, did not inhibit the number of implants at all. When the Zoapatle was prepared from *Montanoa tomentosa* it did not alter the normal structural changes of the uterine by days 5 and 8 of pregnancy in the rat. On the other hand, Zoapatle made from *Montanoa frutescens* caused profound alterations on those structures. These included loss of epithelial lining, thickened blood vessels and alterations in endometrial stroma cells. These morphological changes fit in with the anti-implantation effect found with experimental administration of Zoapatle. The chemical basis of this activity is starting to be found. A number of unique biochemicals are being found, such as kaurenoic acid, kauradienoic acid (its mixture), zoapatanol and montanol. Kaurene compounds appear to be several times more potent than montanol and zoapatanol in their activity on the uterus.

A review of recent published material reveals many patents dealing with the isolation, characterisation and total synthesis of some of Zoapatle's constituents. Clearly this Mexican herb is being seen by both scientists and the drug industry as potentially a new, safe, reliable, inexpensive and profitable contraceptive agent.

The People's Republic of China is at the forefront of this field of herbal reseach. Chinese scientists have capitalised on the rich flora and the ethnomedical experience in China in their pursuit of fertility-regulating agents from natural products. Discoveries range from anti-implantation agents to abortifacient and pregnancy-terminating compounds, as well as a male contraceptive. Much of the excellent research is filled with a quality of social concern and relevance that Western institutions could benefit from. It is to be hoped that further research and collaboration of this quality will take place to help solve the problem of the population explosion.[17]

Ayurvedic medicine from the Indian sub-continent is suggesting important leads for researchers in this field.

Ancient Indian literature abounds with information on large numbers of plants reputed to have sterilising, contraceptive and abortifacient properties. Scholars of Ayurveda have also mentioned several plants in their Ayurvedic treatises. A number of these preparations are still being used by Ayurvedic physicians all over India, who claim their effectiveness but are unable or unwilling to produce data.

A herbal remedy with an ancient history is currently receiving attention as a potential tool in population control. *Hibiscus rosa sinensis* is a common ornamental plant cultivated widely throughout India and Burma. Flowers of this plant are said to possess anti-fertility property by ancient Ayurvedic texts. It is traditionally used in Kerala (Southern India) for its emmenagogue and contraceptive action.

The flowers appear to have a post-coital anti-fertility activity. A study undertaken in 1976 indicated that they possess significant anti-fertility activity with the effects dependent upon the dose, duration of the treatment and the stage of the pregnancy. An anti-fertility agent can work by any one or combination of factors. These can include: rapid expulsion of the fertilised ova from the fallopian tube or by some tube-locking mechanism; as a blastocyst-toxic agent; by the inhibition of implantation due to a disturbance in estrogen–progesterone balance; or through foetal absorption or abortion, perhaps due to lack of supply of nutrients to the uterus and thus to the embryo.

In the light of these observations, it seems probable that the maximum anti-fertility activity occurs through some inhibition of implantation. A restriction of oestrogen levels, which is indispensable for implantation, is considered a probable cause in termination of pregnancy, as the herbal extract possesses potent anti-estrogenic property. It seems probable that the herb alters, in one way or other, the delicate estrogen–progesterone balance, resulting in termination of pregnancy.[18]

However, not only does *H. rosa sinensis* have an impact on female reproduction but also on that of males. Extracts of the flowers also affect the generation of sperm as well as the endocrine function of the testes themselves. This

41

may be due to the inhibition of synthesis or the release of gonadotropins from the pituitary gland, a direct inhibitory effect of testes or hormonal activity. The extract causes a reduction in the weights of the testes, other reproductive organs and the pituitary gland, along with a decrease in levels of the gonadotrophin hormones. After stopping the administration of the herb, spermatogenesis and secretory activity of accessory sex organs started again, indicating that the effects are transient.

Hormonal activity is a totally integrated process, so it is important to look at any possible wider endocrine impact. The thyroid and adrenal are apparently unaffected, suggesting that the inhibitory effects on spermatogenesis are selective, mediated via the pituitary gland, without affecting pituitary-adrenal and pituitary-thyroid function.

Though effective in affecting spermatogenesis, the herb's use as a male contraceptive is unlikely due to an associated reduction of libido because it suppresses endocrine activity of the testis. Although the effects are reversible, persistent daily therapy would be needed because of the rapidity by which pituitary function could recover. Such a herbal remedy, having a potent anti-fertility activity in women and reversible anti-spermatogenic effect in men, offers the potential of a safe and acceptable aid in the drive to controlling population growth.

PLANTS AND CANCER RESEARCH

Herbal remedies have a long and honourable history in the treatment of cancer. It will surprise many people that they are still at the core of modern medicine's fight against this intransigent disease. From the perspective of holistic medicine, any approach to cancer must take into account the whole of the person's life and not simply be a matter of destroying the tumour. A deep process of healing and re-evaluation is essential. Exploration of this approach is beyond the remit of this book but, as anti-tumour herbs are considered, remember that their use has to be incorporated into a broad treatment of the whole person.

The orthodox chemotherapeutic approach to cancer is based upon drugs that inhibit the characteristically uncontrolled development of abnormal cells. This is done either by inhibiting cell division or by killing the cells. Many of the chemicals used are based upon chemical-warfare agents such as nitrogen mustard gas. It was discovered that when used in a controlled therapeutic way the toxicity could be directed to some degree. The ideal chemotherapeutic drug would kill the cancer cells without damaging normal cells. Drugs based upon the chemical attack of alkylating agents such as nitrogen mustard have not proved all that successful in being both effective against cancer cells while harmless to others.

Research is focusing on the search for new molecular prototypes, new types of chemotherapeutic agent, and plant medicines are proving to be excellent sources of these new compounds. While herbalists know well that plants have much to offer in the treatment of cancer, it is coming as a surprise to researchers that our 'weeds' have such virtues. A recent survey lists over 1,400 genera of herbs that have a history of use in cancer treatments.[19,20] The research is showing a chemical basis for the reputation of well-known anti-cancer remedies, as well as suggesting exciting possibilities in 'new' plants.[21] This search for novel anti-cancer drugs is paradoxically producing excellent scientific information on many previously unresearched herbal remedies.

Of the worldwide efforts being made, perhaps the best known is that under the auspices of the United States National Cancer Institute. The rationale of their programme is the screening of all the flowering plants of the world to identify anti-tumour activity. This shows a fundamental assumption that herbal medicines have a positive role to play in the healing arts. A project of this type is a major undertaking, when it is remembered that an estimated 500,000 species exist worldwide. Over 30,000 plants have been tested since the programme began in the late 1950s. Between 3,000 and 4,000 plant samples from approximately 2,000 species are tested each year. Wherever possible, different parts of the same remedy are examined.

Almost 10 per cent of the plants tested show positive results in the anti-tumour tests used. The techniques and findings are described in the references.[22] In other words, many hundreds of potentially useful chemicals have been found so far, even with under 10 per cent of the plants yet examined. This begs the question of the validity of using the plants themselves, as the research does not examine the use of the whole plant on human cancers. The evidence would justify such research.

HERBALISM, ART AND SCIENCE

From this very compressed review it is apparent that a group of secondary plant products such as the terpenes or saponins have a great impact on human physiology. While the therapeutic implications are obvious, an all-too-common mistake is to view these findings as simply those of interesting drugs from plants. There are lessons to be gleaned here concerning the integration of plant and human biochemistry. The use of whole plants cannot any longer be ignored by the medical profession on the grounds of lack of research or inefficacy.

A common complaint from pharmacologists is the apparent toxicity of plant-derived drugs that makes them inappropriate for human use. This is often a by-product of the chemical's being taken out of context of its bio-evolved milieu. An example of such blinkered research is an alkaloid found in *Camptotheca acuminata* that has marked anti-tumour and anti-leukaemic activity in the laboratory. Great hopes were raised for camptohecin as a potential cancer treatment, regrettably dashed when the high toxicity of the drug became apparent. However in the literature no reference is made to work on the whole plant.[23] Whole plants usually have physiologically potent chemicals buffered in a safe chemical matrix. This is a concept alien to pharmacology where the emphasis is on purified, accurate dosages of specific chemicals. Herbalism is an imprecise art as well as a science.

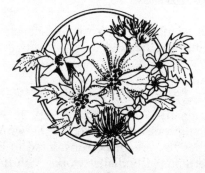

3 · HOW TO CHOOSE THE RIGHT HERB

There is nothing inherent in a plant that defines the way it should be used, and with the wealth of herbs on this planet, some coherent selection criteria are essential to guide herbalists in their healing work. Over half a million plants present themselves as possible healing remedies. The British medical herbalist routinely uses 250, while in China the herbal practitioner has about 2,000 easily available in community pharmacies. Some set of guidelines is obviously being applied to whittle down 500,000 to a more manageable figure, but what are they?

There are a number of useful ways to group the relevant criteria, but three categories are most helpful in Western herbalism.

- Assessment of the herb's impact upon the body and mind. This is a plant-orientated category.
- Using herbs within the context of a system of some kind. This is a person-orientated category.
- Non-therapeutic criteria such as aesthetics, economics and ecology.

Applying these three sets of criteria facilitates the formulation of treatments that can be wholly specific for an individual's unique needs while being environmentally sensitive and economically reasonable. Each of these will be considered in depth.

ASSESSMENT OF THE HERB'S IMPACT

The herbal remedies of the world vary in strength from potentially lethal poisons, if taken at the wrong dosage, to gentle remedies that might be considered to be foods. The holistically orientated herbalist works with the underlying idea that the body is self-healing and that the therapist simply supports this innate healing process. Thus the tonic herbs become of paramount importance as this is exactly what they do. A characteristic of tonics is that they are all gentle remedies that have a mild yet profound effect upon the body. Not all herbal remedies are tonics, of course, with many having a powerful impact upon human physiology. These must be used with the greatest respect, their use being reserved for those times of illness where strong medicine is called for.

By identifying the intensity of impact upon an individual, a useful selection criterion is found. The remedies may be categorised in the following way:

1. *Normalisers* – these are remedies that nurture and nourish the body in some way that supports inherent processes of growth, health and renewal. These are the tonics and are often seen as herbal foods. The Nettle, Cleavers and Chickweed are excellent examples.
2. *Effectors* – these are remedies that have an observable impact upon the body. They provide humanity with the herbs used in the treatment of the whole range of human illness. They can in turn be divided into two groups depending upon how they work:

- *Whole-plant actions*, where the effects are the result of the whole plant impacting the human body. An example would be anti-microbial remedy Echinacea or the anti-inflammatory herb Meadowsweet. Actions are discussed in more depth below.
- *Specific active chemicals*, where the effect is the result

of a chemical whose impact is so overpowering upon the human body that whole-plant effects are not usually seen. Due to the presence of such intense chemicals they are potentially poisonous if taken at the wrong dose or in the wrong way. The cardio-active herb Foxglove and the Opium Poppy are good examples.

The value of tonic herbs lies in their normalising, nurturing effects. These invaluable remedies will usually have some associated action that will further indicate their best use. The cardiovascular tonic Hawthorn is an excellent example that tones the whole system while specifically dilating blood vessels and lowering elevated blood pressure. Whenever possible, the herbalist will focus on the use of such remedies, and will use stronger effectors only if absolutely necessary. The chemically based effectors are hardly used at all. They are, however, the foundation of modern allopathic medicine.

The tonics can play a specific role in ensuring that the individual is at his or her personal peak of health and vitality. The quality of such a state of well-being will vary from person to person, but everyone will sense an improvement in their general experience of life. Tonics may also be used specifically to ward off a known health problem or a family weakness. Each system of the body has plants that are particularly suited to it, some of which are tonics. By selecting remedies that act as tonics for the different systems of the body, it is possible to do some impressive preventative work. With the following list, always take into account the broader picture of a herb's range of actions, as it needs this breadth of vision to enable a coherent choice to be made.

- *Cardiovascular* – Hawthorn and Garlic. The bioflavonoid containing herbs such as Ginkgo, Buckwheat and Lime Blossom are especially useful for strengthening blood vessels.
- *Respiratory* – Mullein, Elecampane and Coltsfoot.
- *Digestive* – No one herb will be an all-round tonic as the system is so varied in its form and functions. The bitter tonics will often be helpful in preventative approaches in health. Examples are Gentian, Agrimony

and Dandelion root. Chamomile and Meadowsweet are so generally helpful to the digestive process that they might be considered as general tonics here.

- *Liver* – Bitter tonics, hepatics and especially Milk Thistle.
- *Urinary* – Bearberry and Corn Silk are very useful.
- *Reproductive* – For women consider Raspberry Leaves, False Unicorn Root and other uterine tonics, while for men Saw Palmetto, Damiana or possibly Sarsaparilla.
- *Nervous* – Oats, Skullcap, St John's Wort, Vervain and Mugwort are all excellent tonic remedies. Siberian Ginseng and Panax Ginseng have a toning effect when the person is under stress because of their effect upon the adrenal glands.
- *Musculo-skeletal* – Celery Seed, Bogbean and Nettles will help prevent any systemic problems manifest as disease in this system. Comfrey and Horsetail will help strengthen the bones and connective tissue.
- *The skin* – Cleavers, Nettles, Red Clover and most of the alterative remedies will help.
- *Infection* – Garlic, Echinacea, and system-specific anti-microbials such as Bearberry for the urinary system.

Since the very beginnings of medicine there has been a striving to make sense of the human body, the ills that assail it and the healing remedies used to treat it. This has led to many models or systems of medicine, most of which are only found now in texts on the history of medicine. The use of herbs has been repeatedly organised and then reorganised into systems that reflect the prevailing world view of the time and culture.

Today is no exception, especially with the herbal renaissance in full flood and the transformation of society and its world view still in mid-process. It is possible to identify a number of commonly found approaches being used currently. There are those that use traditional knowledge or work within the framework of an existing philosophical system. The first grouping based upon the world's folk traditions varies depending upon the tradition used, and the examples of the second group differ depending on the philosophy at their core. The philosophical context may be one of the profoundly holistic systems of Asia or the Western approach which is based on what has been called the biomedical model. This Western model does not mean that the herbs must be used within a disease-centred approach to medicine, but rather should be used within a holistic context.

TRADITIONAL USES

Traditional folk use of herbal remedies is familiar to everyone in some form or another. This is the way in which information about herbal usage has been from generation to generation, but it is also this empirical and unquestioning use that gives herbalism a bad name among the scientific community. Their loss! Folk wisdom is of inestimable value and relevance. Generations of experience and accrued insight are not to be taken lightly. As an example, consider that it is this very folk knowledge from around the world that is often pointing the way in the pharmacologist's search for new and powerful medicines. The use of Wild Yam (*Dioscorea spp.*) as a source of hormone precursors and the Madagascan Periwinkle (*Canthareus spp.*) for anti-leukaemia drugs are examples.

The bulk of the world's health care is still based on the traditional use of local herbal remedies. The relevance of this worldwide traditional folk use is recognised by the World Health Organisation and promoted through their Traditional Medicine programme. All cultures of the world have a herbal tradition. It may be a thriving aspect of their modern life or an apparently more or less moribund historical memory. A visit to any market in Italy will demonstrate the vitality of the herbal tradition there. In contrast, by the early 1970s traditional use of plant medicines appeared to be almost past in Britain. However, with the renewal of interest in herbs as part of a wider re-awakening to the natural world, it was soon discovered that much of the tradition was alive and well. Remedies and recipes for herbal teas had been handed down from generation to generation and are still remembered. The change in social atmosphere regarding herbs has given 'permission' for people to recollect such gems of knowledge.

Wales has a strong modern herbal tradition with clearly recognisable roots in the flowering of Welsh culture in the days of the old princes of Wales. In the rural areas are many people who know one or two herbal combinations that are specific for certain conditions. An often encountered one is an ointment for eczema. They are usually very effective but the people using them rarely know why, and often know no other herbal information. These herbal recipes usually have their origins in the medieval physicians of Myddfai, doctors at the court of the rulers of Wales. These physicians possessed a deep and profound knowledge of herbs and the healing process, well in advance of what was available in England and the rest of non-Islamic Europe at the time.

The continuity of the tradition is paradoxically due to the attempts to destroy the culture that supported the physicians. When the English invaded and conquered Wales, the royal court was destroyed. The knowledge and wisdom of the physicians of Myddfai was in part dispersed throughout the people, in a successful attempt to preserve it. It would appear that certain families were given specific remedies to keep safe and pass on from generation to generation. The recipes and information were never given to anyone outside the family, but the medicine was given freely to anyone who needed it. This wisdom can still be found in the hills and valleys of Wales.

Usually, however, folk traditions in the West are vestigial or have been recently revived by well-meaning adherents. This makes changing or developing herbal treatments problematic. Unless the herbalist is part of an actively living tradition, it is unwise to question or change the handed-down knowledge, as the basis of that knowledge is no longer extant. An example may clarify this.

When in practice in west Wales I came across a hill farmer who made an ointment for the treatment of shingles, a painful and intransigent viral infection of nerve ganglia that is experienced as affecting the skin. On two occasions it was observed clearing trigeminal shingles in 3–5 days, a feat that allopathic medicine or modern herbalism would be hard pressed to duplicate. However, the farmer died childless, without imparting the secret recipe, and especially not to an upstart English herbalist from the town!

All attempts to identify the many herbs used failed, apart from one herb out of the whole combination. This was Biting Stonecrop (*Sedum acre*), a herb that is hardly ever used today and which the seventeenth-century herbalist Culpeper insists must not be put in any ointment. Formulation involved using pig's urine as an extraction vehicle. Apart from practical questions about how to collect the urine(!), modern sensibilities and hygiene considerations would probably suggest using water instead. However, from a therapeutic perspective using pig's urine in this way should not be discarded for hygienic reasons alone. When shamans in Siberia were studied in the early twentieth century it was found that during visionary rituals involving the psychoactive fly agaric mushroom (*Amanita muscaria*), they would drink their own urine. This lengthened and deepened the experience because there are metabolites of the alkaloid muscimole present which are also psychoactive. Is it not possible that some complex process between herbs and pig's urine produced an antiviral metabolite that was absorbable through the skin?

Although this might sound far-fetched, there is no denying that the ointment worked. Unless one knows why something is in the mixture, can it be taken out without losing the desired effect? If the recipe is changed in that way the formulation is no longer the traditional one.

As fundamentally valuable as traditional folk knowledge is, it has limited application within modern holistic herbal practice. The use of herbal remedies in this way, relating specific plants to a specific disease or symptom, is little more than what we may call 'organic drug therapy'. Simply using remedies for such symptomatic relief ignores all the insights of holistic medicine. The ancient folk traditions of the world provide a wonderful foundation upon which the medical

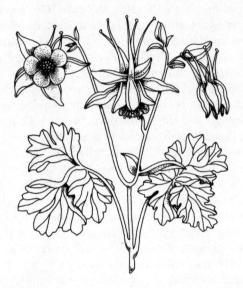

Figure 3   *Columbine*

herbalist may build the holistic herbalism of the future.

PHILOSOPHICAL SYSTEMS

Medical herbalism has most to offer to holistic medicine when used within the context of a coherent philosophical system. Such systems work with intellectual, conceptual models of what a human being is and also what the disease process is. This description of health and human wholeness is simply a subset of that culture's model of the nature of the world itself. These systems may be an overly reductionist interpretation of the biomedical model of Western medicine or the more holistic medical systems of China and India.

Perhaps the best-known of such philosophical systems that are still thriving in the face of the intellectual imperialism of Western medicine are traditional Chinese medicine, Ayurveda and Unani medicine. Other systems are those of cultures such as Japan, Korea and Ghana, or where herbal medicine is integrated into approaches to spirituality and transformation, as in the anthroposophical vision of

Rudolf Steiner. The techniques of any medical system are an expression of its ideas and theories. These in turn are a specific development of the philosophy of the culture concerned. Thus traditional Chinese medicine (TCM) is an application to medicine of a Confucian/Taoist world view. Similarly Ayurveda is an expression of the profound perspectives that come from Hindu experience and spirituality.

It is important that the world view within which any medical practitioner is working be clearly acknowledged and expressed, as this perceptual and contextual environment colours all that occurs and may either limit or facilitate the healing work undertaken. Health care does not happen in a philosophical vacuum, but within a context of a world view and belief system, and if not articulated overtly then it will be implied by default. A problem of subtle cultural chauvinism often arises when comparisons between the different health-care systems of the world is made. In the discussion that follows no value judgements are being made, simply an exploration of practical considerations for both practitioner and patient in the West.

The ancient medical systems of the world are profoundly holistic in both diagnosis and therapeutics, a direct result of their focused expression of spiritually whole and integrated cultural world views. This is often the attraction for Western herbalists, but also paradoxically the primary stumbling block! The holistic strengths of such non-reductionist systems appears to fulfil the deep need experienced by Western practitioners for a holistic approach that is meaningful, practical and relevant.

This confronts the Westerner with some immediate drawbacks. For the therapeutic benefits inherent in these systems to be harvested, the practitioner should ideally be at home in the underlying world view of the culture that gave it birth. In TCM, the names of organs and elements are translated as their English equivalents, but their meaning is different: not a mistranslation, but very different concepts. TCM does not perceive the brain as an organ, and puts the focus of therapeutic work on balancing the flow of *chi* within the body. Disease is seen as an indicator of underlying processes rather than the focus of treatment. The Western practitioner drawn to TCM or Ayurveda must embrace the personal implications for change and transformation inherent in that system.

When this is done then the therapeutic relationship between patient and practitioner can be truly holistic because the therapist is coming from a place of personal integration and harmony. TCM is an expression of seeing and experiencing the world in ways that are different to the Western stance, and when it is used out of context of the deeper world view, the transformative possibilities of healing become severely limited, and the antithesis of holistic medicine. There is no need for the patient to become a Confucian though! TCM is a powerful and effective therapy that has much to offer our suffering culture.

Recognising the fundamental role played by such all-encompassing cultural perspectives highlights the need for a Western context for holistic medicine. Acceptance of the biomedical model as a useful intepretation of the body does not then mean that the analytical and reductionist approach that characterises modern medicine in the West is the only option. There is a dawning recognition of the possibilities that arise if the biomedical model is used as a basis for treating the whole person and not simply the disease.

This also leads to the experience of frustration that plagues Western health-care professionals when they initially explore holistic medicine. There is yet to be written a definitive text on Western holistic medicine, a guide for the practitioner that clearly illuminates these new and exciting perspectives. Although there is a veritable maelstrom of activity among holistic practitioners, exploring and applying the new ideas, it is still early days.

For some this is just too frustrating, leading to an abandonment of the endeavour or a turning to one of the oriental systems. For others this is a very exciting time to be involved in medicine. The unclarity of the situation is one aspect of a flowering of new ideas. There is no textbook because the ideas have not reached the stage where they can be written in stone. It is a time of flux, where many new insights are being obtained and old ideas are being reassessed and discarded or embraced anew. While there may be no clear holistic context yet defined for Western medicine, many of the different approaches in the wide field of health care have achieved much in that direction.

Herbal medicine has a unique contribution to make in this time of change. As a healing modality it is inherently holistic in that its very nature is ecological. The use of plants links both patient and practitioner into their environment in profound ways, facilitating a healing process that could be seen as therapeutic ecology. Such a herbal contribution is but one part of the mosaic that will be Western holistic healing.

The medical herbalist uses a model that enables a prescription to be formulated that addresses the needs of the whole person. The herbal component must be used in the context of addressing non-herbal factors such as diet, lifestyle, emotional, mental and spiritual factors, all of which must take place in the context of their socio-economic context. Such a model provides the practitioner with the possibility of identifying and addressing a whole range of factors, from symptoms and disease pathology to constitution and whole-body toning.

A MODEL OF HOLISTIC HERBAL MEDICINE

This model is not new but rather a formulation of well-established and proven approaches described in holistic terms. There is little that is truly new in such an ancient field as herbalism! The model is applied to the patient's unique needs following skilled diagnosis by a well-trained medical herbalist. Specific examples are explored elsewhere in the book. It is based upon a five-stage process:

- herbal actions;
- system affinity;
- specific remedies for the illness;
- herbal biochemistry;
- intuition.

Herbal actions describe the ways in which the remedy affects human physiology. Plants have a direct impact on physiological activity and by knowing what body process you want to help or heal, the appropriate action can be selected. Obviously selection of actions that are suitable for a specific person will depend on accurate diagnosis. A range of these actions are described below.

Some herbs show an *affinity* for certain organs, body systems or even specific types of tissue. They work as specific tonics or nutrients for the areas involved. Many herbs can be used freely and safely as part of one's lifestyle without thinking of them as 'medicines'. They are at their best when used to nurture health and vitality, so preventing health problems arising. During illness the system-affinity herbs will enhance the general health of the organ or system concerned when combined with remedies selected for their specific actions. They are especially useful where a tendency towards illness is recognised but no overt disease is present. Using herbs in this way opens the possibility of overcoming a weakness that could lead to disease later in life.

The wealth of herbal knowledge that has been garnered over many generations is rich in plants that are traditionally *specific* in the treatment of certain diseases or symptoms. While holistic healing aims at going beyond symptomatic therapy, this knowledge deserves great respect. Knowledge of specific remedies that may heal their illness can add much to a prescription based on appropriate actions and system support.

Increasing attention is being given to the *biochemistry* of herbal active constituents. This has led to the development of many lifesaving drugs, but is very limited as an approach to using whole plants. In the hands of an experienced herbalist, knowledge of plant pharmacology can add to the healing possibilities, but not as much as is often thought.

There is a flowering of *intuitive* rapport between herbalists and their plants. Intuition has a special role to play in healing, and the unique relationship between plant and person augments it well. It is rarely possible to set things up so that such insightful intuition always flows, but when it does it should be embraced. Intuitive knowledge should always be checked if at all possible. For example, if a practitioner is not clear on the difference between Bearberry, Barberry and Bilberry it might lead to unfortunate misunderstanding!

THE ACTIONS OF HERBS

A great deal of pharmaceutical research has gone into analysing the active constituents of herbs to find out how and why they work. A much older, and far more relevant approach is to categorise herbs by looking at what kinds of problems can be treated with their help. In some cases the action is due to a specific chemical present in the herb (as in the anti-asthmatic effects of Ma Huang) or it may be due to a complex synergistic interaction between various constituents of the plant (the sedative Valerian is an example). However, it is best to view the actions as an attribute of the herb as a whole, and any understanding of the chemistry as simply an aid in prescription. The application of the insights offered by the actions approach is explored in the next chapter.

Adaptogens They increase resistance and resilience to stress, enabling the body to avoid reaching collapse because it can adapt around the problem. An inability to cope with external pressures leads to many health repercussions. Adaptogens appear to work through support of the adrenal glands.

Alteratives Herbs that gradually restore proper functioning of the body, increasing health and vitality. Some alteratives support natural waste elimination via the kidneys, liver, lungs, or skin. Others stimulate digestive function or are anti-microbial, while others just work!

Anti-catarrhals Anti-catarrhals help the body remove excess catarrhal, whether in the sinus area or other parts of the body. Catarrh is not in itself a problem, but when too much is produced it is usually in response to an infection or as the body's way of removing excess carbohydrate.

Anti-inflammatories They soothe inflammations or reduce the inflammatory tissue directly. They work in a number of different ways, but rarely inhibit the natural inflammatory reaction as such; rather they support and encourage the work the body is undertaking.

57

Anti-microbials   Anti-microbials help the body destroy or resist pathogenic micro-organisms. They help the body strengthen its own resistance to infective organisms and throw off the illness. While some contain chemicals which are antiseptic or specific poisons to certain organisms, in general they aid the body's natural immunity.

Anti-spasmodics   Anti-spasmodics ease cramps in muscles. They alleviate muscular tension and, as many are also nervines, ease psychological tension as well. There are anti-spasmodics that reduce muscle spasming throughout the body, and also those that work on specific organs or systems.

Astringents   Astringents have a binding action on mucous membranes, skin and other tissue. It is due to chemicals called tannins, named after their use in the tanning industry. They have the effect of precipitating protein molecules, thus reducing irritation and inflammation, creating a barrier against infection that is helpful in wounds and burns.

Bitters   Herbs with a bitter taste, having a special role in preventative medicine. The taste triggers a sensory response in the central nervous system. A message goes to the gut releasing digestive hormones leading to a range of ramifications including: stimulation of appetite; a general stimulation of the flow of digestive juices; an aid to the liver's detoxification work and an increase of bile flow and also stimulation of gut self-repair mechanisms. All of this from a nasty taste in the mouth!

Cardiac remedies   This is a general term for herbal remedies that have a beneficial action on the heart. Some of the remedies in this group are powerful cardio-active agents such as Foxglove, whereas others are gentler, safer herbs such as Hawthorn and Motherwort.

Carminatives   Plants that are rich in aromatic volatile oils stimulate the digestive system to work properly and with ease, soothing the gut wall, reducing any inflammation that might be present, easing griping pains and helping the removal of gas from the digestive tract.

Demulcents   Herbs rich in mucilage that soothe and protect irritated or inflamed tissue. They reduce irritation down the whole length of the bowel; reduce sensitivity to potentially corrosive gastric acids; help to prevent diarrhoea and reduce the muscle spasms which cause colic; ease coughing by soothing bronchial tension and relax painful spasm in the bladder.

Diaphoretics   They promote perspiration, helping the skin eliminate waste from the body, thus helping the body ensure a clean and harmonious inner environment. Some produce observable sweat, while others aid normal background perspiration. They often promote dilation of surface capillaries, so helping improve poor circulation. They support the work of the kidney by increasing cleansing through the skin.

Diuretics   Diuretics increase the production and elimination of urine. In herbal medicine, with its ancient traditions, the term is often applied to herbs that have a beneficial action on the urinary system. They help the body eliminate waste and support the whole process of inner cleansing.

Emmenagogues   Emmenagogues stimulate menstrual flow and activity. In most herbals, however, the term is used in the wider sense of a remedy that normalises and tones the female reproductive system.

Expectorants   Strictly speaking these are herbs that stimulate removal of mucous from the lungs, but often mean a tonic for the respiratory system. Stimulating expectorants 'irritate' the bronchioles causing expulsion of material. Relaxing expectorants soothe bronchial spasm and loosen mucous secretions, helping in dry, irritating coughs.

Hepatics   Hepatics aid the liver. They tone, strengthen and in some cases increase the flow of bile. In a broad, holistic approach to health they are of great importance because of the fundamental role of the liver in the working of the body.

Hypotensives   Plant remedies that lower abnormally elevated blood pressure.

Laxatives   Laxatives stimulate bowel movements. Stimulating laxatives should not be used long term. If this appears to be necessary then diet, general health and stress should all be closely considered.

Nervines Nervines help the nervous system and can be meaningfully subdivided into three groups. Nervine tonics strengthen and restore the nervous system. Nervine relaxants ease anxiety and tension by soothing both body and mind. Nervine stimulants directly stimulate nerve activity.

Rubefacients They generate a localised increase in blood flow when applied to the skin, helping healing, cleansing and nourishment. They are often used to ease the pain and swelling of arthritic joints.

Tonics Tonics nurture and enliven. Truly gifts of Nature to a suffering humanity – whole plants that enliven whole human bodies, gifts of the Mother Earth to her children. To ask how they work is to ask how life works!

Vulneraries Remedies that promote wound healing. Used mainly to describe herbs for skin lesions, the action is just as relevant for wounds such as stomach ulcers.

NON-THERAPEUTIC CRITERIA

Applying the therapeutic criteria described above may sometimes lead to a list of equally relevant remedies. To help further in the selection process there are a number of non-therapeutic factors that can be taken into account. These are aesthetic, economic and environmental.

AESTHETIC CRITERIA

There is no reason for herbal medicines always to taste unpleasant! When the choice arises take into account taste, aroma and visual appeal. These factors are a matter of personal taste, but it is fine to select from the list of herbs that results from applying therapeutic criteria based upon personal aesthetic preference. The only general exception is bitter herbs. If bitterness is indicated, then they must be tasted, otherwise the healing value is lost.

An example is a cough remedy widely used in France. This is composed of the flowers of herbs that ease the cough reflex and help remove phlegm from the lungs. It is straightforward to make a herbal cough mixture that works well, but such effective combinations are often composed of acrid or unpleasant-tasting plants. The same therapeutic results are achieved with the flower mixture, but in addition there is a wonderful aroma, a delicate taste and beautiful colour.

ECONOMIC CRITERIA

Ideally herbs should be free of charge. Nature does not impose a financial levy on herbs as they grow wild and free. There may be environmental costs to take into account, but that is another matter. When the choice arises use common and inexpensive herbs. Expensive, rare or imported plants may not be any better in a particular case than common and not very glamorous Nettles or Cleavers. The fast-developing herb industry has a financial stake in the promotion of expensive 'new wonder herbs' from exotic parts of the world. Just remember that Milton Keynes or Hoboken are exotic locales to most of the world!

ENVIRONMENTAL CRITERIA

Seeing ecological relationships as having a bearing on the healing arts can lead to some important broader implications. The choice of most relevant therapy should be based on the needs of the individual concerned; however, Donne's insight that 'no man is an island' becomes crucial here. In a world where human impact has become life-threatening, the broader implications of health practices must be taken into account. If the ecological effects of drug therapy or herbal therapy are compared, a vital selection criterion reveals itself.

From the Gaian perspective it is problematic to talk of chemical drugs as unnatural and herbal remedies as natural. The integration between plants and humanity on the bio-chemical level shows that chemistry is also 'natural'. If a chemical exists in the body of Gaia it must be natural, if it was not it could not exist without causing major trauma to life on Earth. This is, of course, the case with technological aberrations such as plutonium, but in general, how can we differentiate what is and isn't natural simply on how it is presented to us? The real problem is how we use the chemistry of nature safely.

In addition to the range of criteria described above, it is possible to use environmental impact as one of the ways of identifying appropriate or inappropriate treatments. An example should clarify this. In the treatment of gastric ulceration a whole spectrum of options are available. A holistic approach will focus not only on treating the stomach itself, but examining diet, lifestyle, general health and so on. Treatment may combine possible food changes, relaxation, exercise, counselling etc. with any specific medicines indicated. How should these medicines be chosen? Herbal remedies have much to offer in the treatment of digestive problems in general, and with ulceration especially, and are arguably more clinically effective than drug therapy. However it is the environmental impact rather than therapeutic factors we are concerned with here. In comparing the impact of the drug Tagamet with the herb Marshmallow root, we have two medications that produce equivalent symptomatic relief for the patient.

Chemical drugs would be used that reduce the production of stomach acid and so reduce irritation of the stomach's mucosal lining. Tagamet is a commonly used preparation of the drug cimetidine which inhibits gastric acid and pepsin production in the stomach through blocking histamine receptors. This makes the drug a widely used treatment for duodenal and gastric ulcers. It is now the most prescribed drug in North America, followed by Valium.

Herbal remedies may be selected that soothe the gastric mucosa, reducing the impact of stomach acid, and promoting the healing of ulceration. Plants that are demulcent, vulnerary and antacid are the most relevant, with the inclusion of nervines to reduce excessive vagal stimulation. Comfrey, Marshmallow root, Slippery Elm, Meadowsweet, Chamomile and Marigold may all have a part in treatment. Used in the context of treating the whole picture, herbal treatments of gastric ulceration are extremely effective.

Regardless of their relative therapeutic merits, if their

respective ecological impact is considered a clear picture emerges. Tagamet is manufactured by a process that is notoriously dirty, producing much waste. This waste has to be disposed of, and even with the best environmental will in the world, there is going to be an impact on the environment, but with less than perfect management there will be great and excessive impact, causing both water and air pollution. The impact on local rivers leads to destruction of insect and fish populations and then potentially, through food webs, birds. The water can also have an adverse effect on the soil through irrigation use. The pollutants put into the air will have an effect not only as a contributing factor to acid rain but a direct impact through specific chemicals present, leading to tree damage, soil effects and rain damage to property.

In the development of the drug and fulfilling government safety standards, many laboratory animals are slaughtered. The morality of this fundamental part of modern health care is dubious in the extreme. However it is a necessary evil when dealing with chemical medicine, as the thalidomide tragedy demonstrated.

Industrial production and distribution of the drug is energy-intensive in ways that the resources of the planet cannot support for much longer. The profligate use of non-renewable energy is, of course, an evil of the whole industrial system and not just the fault of Tagamet! There is also the potential for political manipulation with the need for energy to manufacture drugs being cited as a justification for the development of nuclear power. The contradictions in that juxtaposition would be funny if they weren't so frightening.

When using proprietary drugs, the patient and prescriber are at the same time supporting and depending upon the multinational drug companies. The very existence of these vast international corporations raises political, economic and ethical questions that go beyond the confines of this brief review. The patient becomes an unwitting financial supporter of these questionable organisations.

Dis-empowerment becomes a key concept, with the individual's health-care needs being answered by the 'experts', the MD to prescribe and the pharmacist to dispense. This is no criticism of the skill and dedication of these professions to their patients' needs, but a recognition that these same patients have relinquished personal responsibility by handing it over to experts.

Added together, this creates a picture of death, destruction and exploitation in the name of personal health. It is worth seeing the hidden costs of the little tablet as the overall cost of treatment goes way beyond the price of the pills. The cost and impact of such a 'simple' treatment for ulcers includes environmental damage, death and the support of a system that may well be at the centre of much planetary dis-ease.

The dilemma about therapeutic choice raised by these ecological, economic and political considerations might seem daunting. Let Gaia come to the rescue! If herbal remedies are viewed in a similar framework, a very different picture is seen.

Preferably the herb is organically grown, or at least there is the need to cultivate the land and so care for it. This will leave the land at least as well off and hopefully the soil will be nurtured through good organic techniques, which Welsh farmers describe as putting 'heart' back into the soil. Soil structure and stability is becoming a major ecological problem in much of the world. A basic principle in ecology is that the more diverse a system is the more stable it is in the face of environmental perturbation, and organic techniques increase the diversity of soil populations.

Wildcrafted plants, or collecting wild plants in their natural environment, highlight the imperative to preserve the environment as a source of plant and seed, but more importantly for the sake of the environment itself. Herbalism as a therapy is part of a dawning awareness in humanity that life does not existence for our use. Life, our planet, Gaia, all these words and concepts express the wonder of being part of the whole. Herbalism is the therapy of *belonging*.

Within this experience of embracing and being embraced by Mother Earth, it is no wonder that herbal medicine, and in our example Marshmallow, involves no abuse of laboratory animals. The traditional use of Marshmallow is ancient with great knowledge of its use in healing. There is no need to 'prove' this with the genocide of more laboratory animals.

There is little energy consumption in the growing of this herb, and so it is ideal as medicine within a self-sufficient low-impact economy. Even if our society does not yet function this way, we can contribute in the right way with an economically and energetically healing remedy for any ulcers the system generates.

Marshmallow, like other remedies, is produced by small-scale growers, and distributed through channels that support a diversified economic system. It is a perfect example of small being beautiful. Not only are there the benefits of small-scale economic and ecological viability, but this is all producing a medicine that carries all the advantages inherent in herb remedies.

The comparison between the two therapeutically equivalent medicines shows that environmental and political criteria can have a lot to contribute to making choices. Put starkly the choice is between being part of a cycle of death and destruction justified by personal health, or being part of a life-affirming cycle using healing herbs for personal health.

The very process of considering these perspectives is part of the healing of humanity's alienation from our world. As we think so we become. What is it to be?

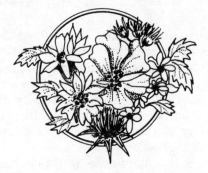

4 · HEALING POSSIBILITIES

The unique contribution of herbal medicine to the healing arts is demonstrated by the way each phase of the unfolding of medicine has embraced herbs as a fundamental component of the newly developed system. Even the flowering of the allopathic approach in the early twentieth century had a fundamentally 'green' core. While herbal practice and therapeutics were largely rejected, the plants themselves became the source of the 'magic bullets' modern medicine is so fond of. Again today, with the new insights and possibilities proffered by holistic medicine, herbalism finds a natural place on the cutting edge of both holistic therapy and theory.

The therapeutic possibilities of herbal medicine in the hands of the skilled professional are at the same time both exciting and challenging. Impressive results are found when herbs are used within the context of one of the holistic models described in the previous chapter, highlighting the invaluable contribution of medical herbalism in the treatment of all human ills. The possibilities become most exciting when using herbalism to augment and nurture that which is 'well'. The deep toning, nutritional and functional support that herbs often provide can support and facilitate the body's undergoing formidable change with relative ease.

A challenge for the medical herbalist is to transcend the conditioned perception and experience of the plants as medicines suited for symptomatic relief only. The alleviation of distress and suffering through addressing symptoms such as pain or inflammation is a vital role for the practitioner to fulfil. The facilitation of an individual's healing process is not simply a matter of easing symptoms, but a deeper process that must address pathology, psychology and even spirituality. In the hands of a practitioner with the personal integrity, insight and vision that embraces such holistic perspectives, herbal remedies can bring about deep and profound physical transformations, enhancing the body's innate striving to heal disease and grow towards health and well-being.

Unfortunately, much modern herbalism remains mired in the allopathic mould that has coloured the whole of medicine for the past sixty years. It can be said that if there is any problem with herbal medicine it is that it works! Too often the practitioner will use herbs to address the surface manifestation successfully while avoiding the challenges of the holistic approach. The patient will experience the removal of symptomatic discomfort and even the 'curing' of their disease, but the profound healing that is the goal of holistic medicine will not occur. Modern herbal medicine must work with deeper factors in a context that is truly holistic. Using the biosphere's wealth of herbal medicines in the broader context discussed below opens possibilities for practitioners of all therapeutic modalities to work with the body and metabolism in a safe, yet profoundly transforming way.

In the following section some examples are explored to clarify these ideas. Approaches to treating the digestive, musculo-skeletal and nervous systems are presented, but this review of therapeutic possibilities is not intended as a self-help guide or therapeutic handbook, but rather as an overview of the vast field. There are many excellent books available on the techniques and practice of herbal medicine, described in the bibliography.

THE DIGESTIVE SYSTEM

Herbal medicine is uniquely suited for the treatment of illness of the digestive system. Throughout the evolutionary process, our food has been our medicine, ensuring that the distinctive healing properties of the herbs have a direct effect upon the lining of the alimentary canal. Not only will there be therapeutic effects due to the metabolism and absorption of the whole range of constituents present in the plant, but there will also be some direct action upon the tissue of the gut through contact. It is the tradition of herbs for aiding digestion that has maintained the strongest foothold in the memory of modern Europe. Whether it be culinary herbs such as Rosemary or as 'medicinal' alcohols like Vermouth or Chartreuse, therapeutic remedies are used in large quantities. The very name Vermouth comes from the bitter remedy Wormwood. Herbs maintain their foothold in the official pharmacopoeias as the major therapeutic agents in the categories of digestive bitters, carminatives and varying strengths of laxatives.

Much digestive-system illness in our society is simply due to abuse. Today's average diet has a preponderance of overly processed foods, a high proportion of chemical additives and the direct chemical irritation of alcohol, carbonated drinks and tobacco. In this context it is easy to see why herbal remedies are so helpful in the various inflammations and reactions that plague such abusers. For example, the direct soothing of herbal demulcents, healing of astringents and general toning of bitters does much to reverse any damage present.

However, as with all true healing, any potential 'cure' lies beyond the range of medicines, whether they be herbal or drug in nature. The healing process must also involve a change of whatever dietary indiscretions are occurring as well as giving attention to lifestyle changes that may be necessary to reduce stress. Herbal medicine can bring about dramatic improvements in even major digestive-system problems but the long-term maintenance of benefit lies in the hands of the person seeking treatment.

Used within such a holistic context, herbal medicine offers specific remedies for particular pathological syndromes and also tonics and normalisers that can help prevent problems manifesting at all. The possibility arises of treating the problem within a context of general nurturing that speeds the improvement in health, enabling a re-establishing of health and harmony. This raises the thorny question again of how these remedies work. Usually there is no adequate answer because no academic research has been undertaken to find a mechanism to explain the clinical findings. As described elsewhere, this may be because no researcher has been interested or funded, or because the complex of factors is so multi-factorial that coherent analysis is almost impossible.

In the hands of a skilled medical herbalist there is much that can be achieved therapeutically, and while each unique individual with, say, a gastric ulcer will have their own array of factors involved, it is possible to identify some useful herbal generalities. A number of herbal actions are of especial value for the digestive system. This is a more helpful way to approach the choice and evaluation of herbal remedies than thinking in terms of specific plants or combinations for certain syndromes, and while there are certain plants that are specific for certain pathologies, these are the exception rather than the rule. Here we shall consider demulcents, bitters and astringents.

DEMULCENTS

A group of herbs that have a wide spectrum of therapeutic use is the demulcent remedies. They are rich in polysaccharide molecules of carbohydrate mucilage, having the physical property of becoming slimy and gummy when in contact with water. This soothes and protects tissue through direct contact. Due to the presence of this mucilage, a number of generalisations can be made about the properties of demulcents:

- they will reduce irritation and inflammation down the whole length of the bowel;

- they diminish sensitivity of digestive-system tissue to corrosive gastric acid and enzymes;
- they may ease the symptoms of diarrhoea;
- they may lessen the muscle spasms that cause colic;
- they reduce coughing due to bronchial irritation;
- they reduce painful spasm in the urinary system.[24]

The last two properties cannot be explained by direct contact between the mucilage and tissues. It has been theorised that the unquestionable clinical findings are based on reflex responses initiated in the gut. The mechanism suggested is based on embryonic developmental associations.

A favourite demulcent remedy among European herbalists is Marshmallow (*Althaea officinalis*). Its traditional and clinical renown, going back to the Egyptians, has recently been confirmed pharmacologically. It was shown in the laboratory to reduce local inflammation by potentiating the action of anti-inflammatory agents released in the tissue itself.[25]

Other remedies that have demulcent action and also have an affinity for the digestive system include Comfrey (*Symphytum officinale*), Plantain (*Plantago major*) and Slippery Elm Bark (*Ulmus fulva*). As will be shown below, the value of these herbs lies in their total range of actions. In addition to Marshmallow's demulcency it also offers anti-inflammatory, diuretic and vulnerary actions. These remedies can be freely used wherever a soothing demulcent is indicated.

BITTERS

Of major importance to the digestive system, as well as the rest of the body, are the bitters. Quite simply these are remedies that have a bitter taste. They affect the tone and functioning of the body as a whole, offering great opportunities to the holistic practitioner. The bitterness is usually described as being due to a 'bitter principle', which may be a volatile oil, an alkaloid, monoterpene iridoids or a sesquiterpene. Absinthin, found in *Artamisias* such as Wormwood, is so bitter it can be tasted at dilutions of 1:30,000!

The physiological activity of all these various chemical varieties appears to be similarly due to a neurological responses triggered by taste receptors in the mouth. Via the central nervous system there is a stimulation of a whole range of digestive activity, the most direct being the secretion of the hormone gastrin. The ramifications of all of this are great indeed. Simplifying for brevity's sake, the responses include:

- a stimulation of appetite;
- a general stimulation of the secretion and flow of digestive juices through the alimentary canal;
- a direct support and stimulation of liver function, especially its detoxification work;
- they help the gut wall repair itself through stimulation of the self-repair mechanisms;
- a general gentle stimulation of endocrine and exocrine activity;
- an effect on the pancreatic hormones that regulate blood sugar;
- a lifting of psychological depression when this is associated with general debility.

Effects occur in a much broader way affecting the healthy activity of the heart and circulation in general.[26] Herbalists have long known of the subtle psychological effects of bitter remedies, as there can be a marked anti-depressive action in some cases as well as a generally tonic effect upon consciousness with remedies such as Mugwort (*Artemisia vulgaris*) and Gentian (*Gentiana lutea*). New research is starting to focus attention of both the clinician and pharmacologist on this use of our herbs.[27]

The therapeutic ramifications of all of this can be quite miraculous. This analytical inquiry is just an attempt to understand the tonic effects of these remedies, effects which go beyond specifics of digestive hormone activity. As digestion and assimilation of food are fundamental to health, bitter stimulation can often fundamentally ameliorate a medical picture that has nothing to do with the digestive process itself.

The remedies available as bitters can range from mild herbs such as Chamomile (*Matricaria sp.*) and Yarrow (*Achillea millefolium*) to quite intense examples such as Wormwood (*Artemisia absinthum*), Gentian and Rue (*Ruta graveolens*). Not only is there a choice of intensity of bitterness but of whatever's the herb's associated actions and system affinity. Consider the strong bitter White Horehound (*Marrubium vulgare*), primarily thought of as an expectorant remedy. This provides the whole range of therapeutic benefits described above while also treating chronic and acute coughs. It makes an ideal remedy where conditions such as bronchitis have been too long standing causing debility and exhaustion. A fair sprinkling of bitter herbs can still be found in the official pharmacopoeias and in current orthodox practice.

ASTRINGENTS

If you have ever had a strong cup of ordinary tea (especially on British Rail) then you have experienced astringency! The tightening of the tissues of the mouth is the proof of the astringent action of the tea plant at work. Astringents are remedies that contain constituents that have a binding action on mucous membranes, skin and other exposed tissue. This is due to a diverse group of complex chemicals called tannins or gallotannins, that have certain chemical and physical properties in common. The name tannin derives from the use they were put to in the tanning industry. They have the effect of precipitating, or curdling, protein molecules. This also happens with starch, gelatin, alkaloids and salts of heavy metals.

This changing of the form of protein is how animal skin is turned into leather, and also what happens with the stewed tea. In other words they produce a kind of temporary leather coat on the surface of the tissue in question. This brings about a number of therapeutic benefits:

• a reduction of irritation on the surface of tissues due to a form of numbing;

72

- a reduction in surface inflammation due to the temporary barrier;
- a barrier against infection is created which is of great help in wounds and burns.

Astringents have a role in a wide range of problems in many parts of the body, but are of great importance in wound healing and conditions of the digestive system. In the intestinal tract they reduce inflammation and inhibit diarrhoea and are widely used in the various diseases of digestion.

Using the insights gained through an understanding of herbal actions can provide a rational and holistic perspective within which to place knowledge of the specific effects of individual remedies. To see the possiblities that open up for the herbalist consider the range of healing actions of Chamomile.

CHAMOMILE

Perhaps the best-known herbal tisane is Chamomile tea, and with such a widely used digestive remedy throughout Europe, its therapeutic use is well documented. The German Chamomile (*Matricaria recutita*) is uniquely suited for digestive problems, combining as it does carminative, anti-spasmodic, anti-inflammatory, antiseptic and gentle bitter actions.[28]

Chamomile has been a valued herb for many thousands of years, with the ancient Egyptians venerating its simple beauty as an embodiment of the Sun. As with many herbs, its modern name can be traced back to the Greeks. The delightful aroma reminded them of apples and the herb was called 'ground-apple', *kamai* (on the ground) – *melon* (apple). In Spanish it is also known as *Manzanilla* or 'little apple'.

There are two herbs which are commonly called Chamomile and used in Western herbalism. Roman Chamomile (*Anthemus nobilis*) is a compact, low-growing perennial plant with tiny daisy-like flowers. The annual German Chamomile (*Matricaria recutita*) is taller and less compact in growth form. They both share the wonderful aroma and although German Chamomile is the preferred medicinal species this is not a rigid rule. Each person will have their own herbal 'allies' and for some people it may well be that Roman Chamomile would be preferable. It has been part of herbal medicine for as long as records exist, and is still very much present in health care, being used wherever it grows in the world. Chamomile is in many pharmacopoeias as an officially recognised medicine, used in orthodox medical practice throughout the continent.

A comprehensive list of Chamomile's medicinal uses would be very long. Included would be insomnia, anxiety, menopausal depression, loss of appetite, dyspepsia, diarrhoea, colic, aches and pains of 'flu, migraine, neuralgia, teething, vertigo, motion sickness, conjunctivitis, inflamed skin, urticaria, etc. This may seem too good to be true, but the whole plant has a wide range of actions in the body. Chamomile is probably the most widely used relaxing nervine herb in the Western world. It relaxes and tones the nervous system, and is especially valuable where anxiety and tension produce symptoms such as gas, colic pains or even ulcers. This ability to focus on physical symptoms as well as underlying psychological tension is one of the great benefits of herbal remedies. Chamomile is safe and effective in all types of stress and anxiety-related problems, and it makes a wonderful late-night tea to help ensure a restful sleep. Throughout Europe it has a reputation as helping with anxious children or even teething infants, where it is used as an addition to the bath. It will also prove helpful to the parents of teething children!

In addition to the direct effect upon the nervous system, Chamomile is also an anti-spasmodic herb. By working on the peripheral nerves and muscle tissue it has an indirectly relaxing effect on the whole body. When the physical body is at ease, ease of mind and heart follows. Chamomile may prevent or ease spasms or cramps in the muscles, such as leg or abdominal cramping. Used as the essential oil added to a bath, it relaxes the body after a hard day while easing the cares and weight of a troubled heart and mind.

Being rich in aromatic essential oil, it acts on the digestive system, gently promoting proper function. This usually involves soothing the walls of the intestines, easing griping pains and helping the removal of gas. It is an effective anti-inflammatory remedy, both internally for digestive and respiratory system inflammations and externally on the skin. A cup of hot Chamomile tea is a simple yet effective way of relieving indigestion, calming inflammations such as gastritis and helping prevent ulcer formation. Using the essential oil as a steam, inhalation will allow the same oils to reach inflamed mucous membranes in the sinuses and lungs. Allopathic medicine places much emphasis on chemicals that work in an anti-inflammatory way to reduce symptoms in many diseases. This symptomatic alleviation is not the way herbal anti-inflammatories should be used, or in fact how they appear to work. Herbs can reduce inflammation in a number of different ways, as discussed elsewhere, but they rarely inhibit the natural inflammatory reaction as such.

Chamomile has a mild anti-microbial action, helping the body to destroy or resist pathogenic micro-organisms. Azulene, one of the components of the essential oil, is bacteriocidal to both *Staphylococcus* and *Streptococcus* infections. As an anti-catarrhal herb, it helps the body remove excess catarrhal build-up in the sinus area, and it may be used in head colds and allergy reactions such as hay fever. Mucus and catarrh are not problems in themselves, they are essential body products, but when too much is produced it is usually in response to an infection, helping the body remove the problematic organism, or as a way of the body's eliminating excess carbohydrate.

In total there is a mild anti-spasmodic effect on smooth muscles that will ease colic, gently sedate and relax the central nervous system, easing the impact of stress, while also supplying an anti-inflammatory effect upon the lining of the digestive system as well as being anti-microbial. There is also a resulting local effect of vasodilation increasing blood flow to the digestive system. This all works together in a way that gives this herb an invaluable role in holistic treatments of many digestive-system diseases, especially where there are associated colic spasms.

This wonderful herb has been a focus of research since pharmacology began. There is a wealth of information about the whole range of its chemical components. However, this does not tell us much about the value and benefits of the herb as used in healing. The activity of the whole plant is always more than the sum of its parts, just as a person is more than the sum of their biochemistry. Herbal medicine treats the unique individual and not just the disease present, and although herbs can be very powerful in addressing symptomology, we limit their potential if we stay at this level. Knowing the chemistry of sesquiterpenes is not the same as knowing Chamomile!

Chamomile essential oil is a unique blend of many individual oils. In addition to a delightful aroma, these oils all have anti-inflammatory, anti-spasmodic, vasodilating and anti-microbial activity in the body. When freshly distilled this beautiful oil is deep blue due to the presence of azulene. Some of the other components of the oil include a range of sesquiterpenes such as α-bisabolol, chamazulene, farnesene and herniarin. Following much pharmacological research, the α-bisabolol has been credited with the ulcer-protective properties of the herb and azulene as the main anti-inflammatory. Important flavonoids have been found that include quercimeritin, which is involved in the reduction of capillary fragility. Apart from the oil there is a bitter principle, flavones, glycosides, salicylic acid, coumarin derivatives and much more. They act as a biologically evolved whole, contributing their specific effects to create a wonderfully rounded digestive remedy.

A review of recent scientific literature shows how much interest this venerable folk remedy is still receiving. Anti-inflammatory effects have been researched in great depth, being the official criteria for its inclusion in many pharmacopoeias. Clinical evaluation in Poland has shown the therapeutic value of toothpaste containing German Chamomile, and a fascinating recent German study demonstrated its efficacy in the healing of wounds caused by tattooing. A common problem with tattoos is a 'weeping' wound where the skin has been abraded. The healing and drying process was compared between patients who were treated with Chamomile and a control group who were not. The decrease of the weeping-wound area as well as the speed of drying was dramatically improved by using Chamomile.[29]

Such research demonstrates statistically what the herbalist knows experientially, that Chamomile will reduce inflammation, colic pain and protect against ulcer formation in the whole of the digestive tract.[30] French researchers found that the extract added during the early stage of Poliovirus development inhibits RNA synthesis in the virus.[31] There are possible new anti-cancer remedies awaiting discovery in this herb. A new sesquiterpene lactone has been isolated from Roman Chamomile which in the laboratory shows a cytotoxic activity at levels that make it worth exploring further.[32]

The value of this wonderful herb is not just as a medicine but as an addition to our lives. As a cosmetic, or in the garden, the beauty of Chamomile shines bright. In Elizabethan England, the herb lawn was a common sight. A wonderful way of cultivating Chamomile is as such a lawn. To quote an old English rhyme:

> Like a chamomile bed
> The more it is trodden
> The more it will spread.

Not only will the herb thrive under foot, each time it is walked upon the aroma will be released. A special way of relaxing with this healing herb for the nervous system is to walk barefoot along a Chamomile lawn when it is moist with morning dew. Just imagine the difference if Wall Street and the Houses of Parliament had Chamomile lawns instead of coffee machines!

Healing is a gift that our world freely gives humanity, a gift that is being rediscovered by our culture at this time of great need, confusion and pain. When many tried and trusted 'answer' seem to cause as much trouble as they solve, nature offers us simple, safe and sound ways to heal.

CLINICAL USE OF HERBS IN GASTRO-INTESTINAL PROBLEMS

Many excellent modern herbals explore treatments for digestive-system problems in some depth.[33] Here we shall only consider some specific therapeutic examples. As the practical details of treatment programmes and how most appropriately to use medicinal plants in the broad context of holistic therapy are beyond the scope of this overview of herbalism, we shall just consider a couple of issues.

Peptic ulceration

The plant kingdom offers much in the way of treatment for this scourge of the modern world. Ulcerative conditions of the stomach, duodenum and oesophagus are very common in our society, with non-prescription symptomatic relief medicines being major money-makers for the pharmaceutical industry. Drug treatment is based primarily upon reducing the corrosive impact of stomach acid on the mucosal lining. This is done through antacid chemicals or other agents that reduce the production in the first place, either directly or indirectly. A holistically orientated practitioner will aim to treat the ulceration in a more deep-seated way. This will often involve dietary advice, psychological counselling and lifestyle re-evaluation. A range of plants are available that appear to work in a broader way to facilitate a reversal of the syndrome present.

Technically these conditions are charactised by a limited ulceration of the mucous membrane that lines the inner wall of the stomach, penetrating through to the muscule coat and occurring in areas exposed to acid and the digestive enzyme pepsin. Gastric ulceration occurs along the lesser curvature of the stomach, while duodenal ulcers are found in the first few centimetres of the duodenum.

Peptic ulcers usually have a chronic, recurrent course, with a variable symptom picture, and in fact only about half of all ulcer patients present to their doctors with the characteristic picture. The pain is often described as burning, gnawing or aching, while the distress is a soreness, empty feeling or'hunger'. This characteristic pain will be relieved by antacids or milk. The typical pain picture in duodenal ulcers is that of hunger pains, while that for gastric ulcers may be brought on by eating.

With the skilled use of plants having demulcent, antacid, astringent and vulnerary actions it is well within the bounds of therapeutic possibilities to bring about a rapid and complete healing of any ulceration. Herbs such as Comfrey (*Symphytum officinalis*), Marshmallow (*Althaea officinalis*), Meadowsweet (*Filipendula ulmaria*), Marigold (*Calendula officinalis*), Chamomile (*Matricaria recutita*) and Golden Seal (*Hydrastis canadensis*) are examples of the remedies that may be used.

The clinical experience of the medical herbalist is now gaining support from research occurring throughout the world. As already pointed out, mucilage is the basis of demulcency and it is this action that is fundamental to any herbal treatment of such stomach conditions. Russian research has found that plant mucilage has a regenerative effect upon the lining of the stomach.[34] They showed that a number of polysaccharides of plant origin exhibited an anti-inflammatory action which compared very favourably to that of the drug butadiene.

Applying the model described above, a number of actions are clearly indicated for the processes behind this disease:

- Demulcents soothe the lining of the stomach, either through a coating or an inherent anti-inflammatory action. Possible herbs include Comfrey, Marshmallow and Slippery Elm.
- Anti-inflammatories will reduce localised mucosal reaction. Possibilities include Chamomile, Meadowsweet and Marigold.
- Astringents will lessen local bleeding. Comfrey and Meadowsweet are especially indicated here.
- Vulneraries speed up natural wound healing. Consider

Comfrey, Chamomile and Golden Seal.

- Carminatives will ease any subsequent flatulence lower down in the abdomen. Chamomile, Peppermint and Valerian are just three possibilities.
- Nervines will help ease background stress involvement. Consider Chamomile, Valerian and Hops as possible remedies.
- Bitters aid the healing process in the latter stages of treatment but are contra-indicated initially because they will stimulate the production of stomach acid and so agravate the problem.
- Alteratives help the body dealing with any systemic problems that might result from the disease.
- Antacids, however, have little to offer other than symptomatic relief.

When considering tonics to supply any appropriate system support, the digestion and subsequent elimination are pivotal, as is the nervous system. Of course any focus of distress or malfunction in any system must be helped. A number of traditional specific remedies will come to mind, but their value is based upon their actions. They include all the remedies mentioned so far.

From this it should be apparent that a number of different herbs and combinations will be effective. The choice of the most appropriate mixture for a specific patient will depend upon the skill of the herbalist. One possible prescription might be the following. A successful herbal component in the treatment of peptic ulceration is a two stage process.

The aim of the first stage is to reduce the accompanying inflammation and initiate healing using demulcents, nervines and vulneraries.

Comfrey root
Marshmallow root
German Chamomile

These herbs will be combined in equal parts as tinctures and a usual dose would be a teaspoonful (5ml) three times a day. Infusion of the fresh or dried herbs may be drunk often to ease symptoms. An infusion of German Chamomile drunk on an empty stomach will help reduce the inflammation and reverse the ulcerative process.

The second stage of treatment aims at toning the recuperating tissue and complete the healing process with a mixture that might include the following herbs:

Golden Seal
Comfrey root
German Chamomile

The addition of Goldern Seal at this stage will speed recovery through its tonic effect upon the mucous membrane lining of the stomach as well as its generalised bitter tonic action. As already pointed out, bitters must not be used while an active ulcer is present.

These mixtures can be adapted to suit a particular individual with their unique factors and needs. If stress and anxiety are major contributing factors then greater emphasis should be placed upon relaxing nervines, such as Valerian or Skullcap. If the herbalist suspects that the liver needs support then possibly Dandelion root may be appropriate. The possible variations are as endless as the variability in people.

All of this herbal therapy must be placed within a broader non-herbal context of treatment. Dietary factors are fundamentally involved in both the causation and treatment of peptic ulceration. As in the other digestive-system conditions discussed so far, all irritant foods must be avoided. Alcohol and tobacco are especially implicated. Pepper, coffee and anything that the patient experiences as a problem should be removed from the diet. Small meals are often better than large meals. Rest and re-evaluation of a lifestyle that may be causing stress is essential.

The liver

Another area of therapy that is particularly well-suited for herbal treatment is that of the liver, both in health and disease. In the unique and often infuriatingly unscientific language of traditional herbalists, much attention is given to 'detoxifying the liver'. The incredible complexity of liver chemistry and its fundamental role in human physiology is so daunting to researchers that the thought that simple plant remedies might have something to offer is both laughable and even insulting to them! However, when these liver remedies have been objectively studied, the findings usually bear out the claims. This again highlights the limiting trap of the current research paradigm.

The liver is a vital organ that fulfils a number of functions within the body. Among these functions, it is the site of carbohydrate metabolism and storage as glycogen; it similarly metabolises both lipids (including cholesterol and certain vitamins) and proteins; it is the place in which bile is manufactured; impurities and toxic material are cleared from the blood; vital blood-clotting factors are produced there and old, worn-out red blood cells are destroyed. Certain reticulo-endothelial cells (the Kupffer cells) play a role in immunity.

While the liver is able to regenerate itself after being injured or diseased, if a disease progresses beyond the tissue's capacity to regenerate new cells, the body's entire metabolism is severely affected. Any number of disorders can affect the liver and interfere with the blood supply, the hepatic and Kupffer cells, and the bile ducts.

From the herbalist's ecological perspective, it is apparent that our evolutionary home – the environment in which we live – will nurture and heal many of the ills of the liver. After all, the liver and its wonderful biochemistry is part of the ecosystem as well. With remedies such as Dandelion (*Taraxacum officinalis*), Balmony (*Chelone glabra*), Fringe-tree Bark (*Chionanthus virginicus*) and the bitter tonics such as Gentian (*Gentiana lutea*), a powerful Materia Medica is available for liver problems. Treatment can range through conditions requiring gentle liver stimulation to even the most profound liver disease. As with most claims made by the medical herbalist, pharmacological and clinical research is starting to support traditional experience and provide a chemical insight into the mechanisms involved.[35] A good example is Milk Thistle.

Milk thistle

The importance of botanical accuracy is highlighted here. In different places this herb is called Milk Thistle, Mary Thistle and even Sow Thistle. To complicate matters the botanical taxonomists have changed the binomial! Milk Thistle is now correctly called *Carduus marianus* and *not Silybum marianus*. In the references that follow this dual nomenclature is unfortunately evident. Historically this herb has been used in Europe as a liver tonic and current phytotherapy indicates its use in a whole range of liver and gall-bladder conditions including hepatitis and cirrhosis. It may also have value in the treatment of chronic uterine problems.

A wealth of research done in Germany is revealing exciting data about reversal of toxic liver damage as well as protection from potential hepatotoxic agents.[36] A number of chemical components of the herb are now being shown to have this protective effect on liver cells. They are all flavones and flavo-lignins, the best studied being silymarin.[37] Silymarin has been shown to reverse the effects of highly toxic alkaloids, such as phalloidine and α-amanitine from the Avenging Angel mushroom (*Amanita phalloides*) as well as also protecting liver cells from the impact of these poisons.[38] The pharmacodynamics, site and mechanism of action of silymarin are becoming well understood, providing insights into the metabolic basis of this herb's activity, an activity long known and used by medical herbalists.

INFLAMMATION AND ARTHRITIS

The plant kingdom abounds with species that act as anti-inflammatories to animal tissue. If the premise is accepted that through an ecological integration most of the biological needs of humanity and the other animals are met by our evolutionary environment, the wealth of anti-inflammatory herbs comes as no surprise. Although they are rarely as immediately powerful as the steroid drugs, they are very rarely as dangerous and potentially life-threatening. It should be remembered that the steroidal anti-inflammatory drugs were developed from plant material and are still largely synthesised from saponins such as diosgenin from the Mexican Yam (*Dioscorea floribunda*).

One of the benefits of modern life is the way in which acute infectious disease has been brought under control. However, in the process there has been a growth of almost epidemic proportions in the chronic degenerative diseases. These cover the whole range of things that can go wrong in the human body, but frequently found symptoms are the pain and discomfort of inflammation. This process is unpleasantly familiar to everyone, and may occur in response to a wide range of traumas from sunburn and wounds, to infection and auto-immune conditions. Whatever the cause, this process is basically the same.

It is characterised by four physical signs: warmth, redness, swelling, and pain. Warmth and redness result from dilation of the small blood vessels in the injured area and increased local blood flow. Because blood vessels become more permeable during inflammation, protein-rich exudate escapes from blood plasma to the damaged tissue and causes swelling. Pain is believed to result from such chemical substances as serotonin or from tension of tissue over the inflamed area. So inflammation in an auto-immune condition such as rheumatoid arthritis is fundamentally the same as that of simple infections or wounds; however, the trigger of the reaction is very different.

Exploring the biochemistry and pathology of this complex process can often imply that chemistry is the medical answer. However, plants used as whole medicines will reduce and soothe much inflammation whether we know the biochemistry or not. The herbs that help the body to combat inflammations are known as anti-inflammatory remedies. Orthodox medicine places much emphasis on chemicals that work in an anti-inflammatory way to reduce symptoms and ease suffering in many diseases, but such symptomatic relief is not the ideal way to use herbal anti-inflammatories. They are safe to use for the relief of pain and discomfort, but offer most when used in combination with other remedies to address the underlying problem.

HERBAL ANTI-INFLAMMATORIES

Herbs can reduce inflammation in a number of different ways but rarely do they inhibit the natural reaction; rather they support and encourage the work the body is doing. An inflammation is a normal body response to infection or other problems, as through localised biochemical and tissue modifications, the inflammatory reaction will often bring about the changes necessary to heal the focus of disease and restore health. It is a mistake to inhibit this response unless it is a life-threatening situation. For example, simply suppressing the symptoms of inflammation in the stomach to relieve the discomfort will not change underlying causes. The alleviation of discomfort could possibly lead to the development of a stomach ulcer because the problem is ignored. We have become conditioned into seeing inflammations as something to suppress and smother, rather than to work with and help. Herbal remedies offer us this possibility, but as in all health matters there is a balance to achieve. Here it is the need to know when an inflammation is one to work with or one to suppress.

Herbal anti-inflammatories fall into four groups depending upon the way in which they work. An understanding of such mechanisms will often provide important clues as to their relevance for different kinds of inflammation. However, it cannot be over-emphasised that the action of any plant is always more than the action of any specific constituent chemical. Keeping this holistic perspective in mind let us look at these groups.

1. Salicin containing

A large range of plants contain natural aspirin-type chemicals called salicylates. It is worth noting that the the whole aspirin group of drugs was originally isolated from plant sources. In fact the name aspirin comes from the old botanical genus name of Meadowsweet (**Spir**aea–**aspir**in), and **sali**cylate derives from Willow's Latin name **Salix**. Those herbs with significant quantities of salicylates have a marked anti-inflammatory effect, without the dangers to the stomach of aspirin itself. In fact Meadowsweet, rich in salicylates, can be used to staunch mild stomach haemorrhage even though the salicylates can cause such problems. Other plants rich in such constituents include Willow Bark (*Salix sp.*), Wintergreen (*Gaultheria*), Birch (*Betula sp.*), many of the Poplars, and Black Haw (*Viburnum prunifolium*). This group is most useful in inflammations of muscles, bones and connective tissue caused by conditions such as osteo-arthritis or sports injuries.

2. Saponin 'steroid pre-cursor' containing

The powerful chemical anti-inflammatories known as steroids were themselves first isolated from plant material and some herbs contain safe-to-use constituents that are metabolised by the body into its own inflammation-fighting steroidal molecules. Such plants will aid in reducing some kinds of inflammation, especially those due to auto-immune problems such as rheumatoid arthritis or Chrohn's disease. Examples are Liquorice (*Glychorriza glabra*) and Wild Yam (*Dioscorea villosa*).

3. Oils

Many of the aromatic herbs with their wonderful essential oils have an anti-inflammatory action. One of the best of these remedies is Chamomile, described in the section on the digestive system. Marigold (*Calendula officinalis*) and St John's Wort (*Hypericum perforatum*) are other well-known plants that contain oils that soothe and reduce inflammation. They work best where the oil can actually make contact with the inflamed tissue as in digestive or skin problems.

4. Other types of anti-inflammatories

As is usual with herbal remedies there are many valuable anti-inflammatories that have no clear cut chemical basis for their action. In some cases it is thought that resins within the herb might be important. This in no way negates their value, rather it shows that there is more to health and well-being than pharmaceutical chemistry! Of the many remedies in this group we can mention Bogbean (*Menyanthes trifoliata*), Devil's Claw (*Harpagophytum procumbens*), Lig-

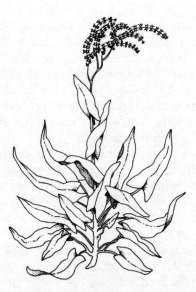

Figure 4   *Sorrel*

num Vitae (*Guaiacum officinalis*) and Black Cohosh (*Cimicifuga racemosa*).

ANTI-INFLAMMATORIES FOR DIFFERENT PARTS OF THE BODY

Each system of the body has plants that are particularly suited to it and additionally work as anti-inflammatory remedies. This allows the herbalist to nurture the health and vitality of a system of the body that is suffering while also reducing any inflammation present. The tonics and herbs with specific affinities come into their own here. The following examples will clarify this.

For the cardiovascular system a number of herbs may be used to reduce inflammations in blood vessels, including Linden Flowers, Hawthorn berries, Horse Chestnut leaves, and Yarrow. They may be used in a range of problems from varicose veins to phlebitis. All these remedies will strengthen the tissue of the system in addition to the soothing anti-inflammatory action. Flavones appear to be very important in this case.

As the herbs go directly to the digestive system they are of especial use in conditions that range from stomach ulcers to colitis and haemorrhoids. Such herbs include Chamomile, Wild Yam, Liquorice, Golden Seal, Marigold and Peppermint. The demulcent remedies, such as Marshmallow, that are rich in mucilage can have a localised effect of reducing inflammation through a contact soothing effect.

A number of herbs soothe the tissue of the urinary system directly as their anti-inflammatory constituents are passed through the kidneys and bladder. Plants that soothe the tissue and reduce infection will also have an anti-inflammatory action. Specific urinary anti-inflammatories are Golden Rod (*Solidago sp.*) and Corn Silk (*Zea mays*).

For the reproductive system, many of the wonderful tonics nature provides for the reproductive process and other specific gynaecological remedies will often act in this way. Lady's Mantle (*Alchemilla arvensis*) and Blue Cohosh (*Caulophylum thalictroides*) are good examples.

For hard-working and abused muscles and bones, the salicylate-containing remedies come into their own. Willow Bark, Meadowsweet, White Poplar and Birch are excellent. Others to consider are Bogbean, Devil's Claw, Black Cohosh, Feverfew (*Chrysanthemum parthenium*) and Wild Yam. The treatment of arthritis conditions responds well to herbal therapy, but works best when done within the holistic perspective of treating the whole person and not simply the 'disease'.

While the nervous system often feels like it needs anti-inflammatories, the best remedies for the 'inflamed state of mind' are the herbal-relaxing nervines. The only true anti-inflammatory for the nervous tissue is St John's Wort, which helps in the recovery of damaged nerves. However, many of the nervines will help such as Oats (*Avena sativa*) and Valerian (*Valerian officinalis*).

There is an abundance of remedies to reduce inflammation on the skin. This is only to be expected if nature does provide us with what we need, considering all the nettles and brambles! A selection of these gifts includes Marigold, St John's Wort, Myrrh (*Commiphora mol-mol*), Golden Seal,

Arnica (*Arnica montana*), Chickweed (*Stellaria media*), and Plantain (*Plantago sp.*).

HERBAL ANTI-RHEUMATICS

All the herbal traditions around the world abound in remedies that are known by the unfortunately vague term of 'anti-rheumatic'. Such a name describes the observed effect but tells nothing about its mode of action. Some well-known examples in the West are:

Angelica	Boneset	Horseradish	Sarsaparilla
Arnica	Burdock	Juniper	White Poplar
Bayberry	Cayenne	Lignum Vitae	Wild Yam
Bearberry	Celery Seed	Meadowsweet	Willow bark
Birch	Cramp Bark	Mugwort	Wintergreen
Black Cohosh	Dandelion	Mustard	Wormwood
Bladderwrack	Devil's Claw	Nettles	Yarrow
Blue Cohosh	Feverfew	Parsley	Yellow Dock
Blue Flag	Ginger	Prickly Ash	
Bogbean	Guaiacum	Rosemary	

These are remedies that have been observed to improve patients' experience of rheumatic problems. That is not to say that they have a specific effect upon the disease or even necessarily upon the musculo-skeletal tissue itself. It is a description of outcome rather than process. The activity of these herbs as anti-rheumatics can be explained as an expression of a more broadly relevant action. This may be due to the main action alone or a more holistic synergy of the plants' total 'actions package'. For example the alteratives can work in a number of different ways as can the anti-inflammatories. Unfortunately this cannot always be worked out.

- *Anti-inflammatories*: Angelica, Celery Seed, Birch, Wild Yam, Meadowsweet, Wintergreen, Lignum Vitae, Devil's Claw, Bogbean, White Poplar, Feverfew, Willow bark
- *Alteratives*: Burdock, Bladderwrack, Lignum Vitae, Devil's Claw, Blue Flag, Bogbean, Yellow Dock, Sarsaparilla, Nettles

- *Diuretics*: Celery Seed, Yarrow, Bearberry, Boneset, Juniper, Parsley, Dandelion
- *Circulatory stimulants*: Horseradish, Mustard, Cayenne, Bayberry, Rosemary, Prickly Ash, Ginger
- *Anti-spasmodics*: Black Cohosh, Cramp Bark
- *Other action or basis unclear*: Arnica, Wormwood, Mugwort, Blue Cohosh

This brief review of anti-inflammatory and anti-rheumatic herbs should illuminate some of the therapeutic possibilities. In the treatment of the plethora of problems that assail the musculo-skeletal system, herbalists have an abundant Materia Medica, allowing the disease process to be addressed from a variety of angles. In the hands of a holistic practitioner this facilitates the flexibility of treatment essential when taking into account individual needs and variability between patients.

ARTHRITIS

Perhaps the most important inflammatory conditions to affect humanity are the many varieties of arthritis and rheumatism, and throughout the world herbal medicine is used in its treatment. Arthritis is a general term for many differently named diseases that produce either inflammation of connective tissues, particularly in joints, or non-inflammatory degeneration of these tissues. The word simply means 'joint inflammation', but because other structures are also affected, the diseases are often called connective tissue diseases. Many of these diseases are characterised by inflammation in the affected tissue. The usual signs of inflammation (warmth, redness, swelling, and pain) are often present.

In some conditions, the inflammation is an immune re-action. This may be the body's defence against invading micro-organisms, but often the immune reaction against the body's own tissue is of unknown cause. The body seems to react against itself rather than against an invading micro-organism. Anti-self antibodies react with intact connective tissue and synovial membranes and thus cause inflammation.

The commonest auto-immune form of arthritis is rheumatoid arthritis. Although the symptoms of rheumatoid arthritis are due to inflammation of the connective tissues, the cause is not at all clear. Characteristically the synovial membranes, or inner linings of the joint capsules, are chronically inflamed. The synovial mass proliferates and thereby destroys cartilage, bone and adjacent structures. Widespread inflammation may involve other tissue leading to painful joints, loss of mobility, and a generalised soreness and depression. Blood tests often reveal the presence of rheumatoid factors, proteins produced by the immune system in response to the rheumatic process.

Utilising a broad holistic approach, herbal medicine works with the whole body promoting an improvement of the condition whilst alleviating pain and discomfort. Simply using anti-inflammatory and anti-rheumatic remedies is not enough; therapy must focus on liver function, circulation, elimination as well as quality of life and experience. We shall consider how a medical herbalist would treat rheumatism and osteo-arthritis.

Rheumatism

This is a notoriously vague and misused description of aches and pains in the musculature of the body. As a common sign of the early stage of many infections and a whole range of auto-immune conditions, careful diagnosis may be called for. As this will often go beyond the usual expertise of the herbalist, a safe guideline is that if symptoms cannot be eased to some degree within a month, consider the problem more deeply.

There are a number of herbal actions indicated for treating the processes behind this disease. The actions mentioned here are explained earlier in the book.

- *Anti-rheumatics* will help through their general value for this body system.
- *Anti-inflammatories* are especially indicated if there is much sensitivity on touch.
- *Alteratives* would be indicated if there is suspicion of a systemic problem.
- *Anti-spasmodics* will ease any associated muscular tension, often the core of this problem.

- *Circulatory stimulants* may help through increasing local circulation; however they are usually best used in the form of rubefacients.
- *Rubefacients* will stimulate circulatory activity, and so promote removal of tissue waste and local supply of oxygen and nutrients.
- *Analgesics* are of limited symptomatic use only.
- *Diuretics* appear to be very effective in easing vague 'rheumatic' aches and pains.
- *Nervines* will help if there is much stress or tension in the person's life.

One of the strengths of medical herbalism is the possibility of supporting a whole range of normal body processes while also focusing on the problematic pathology. In such an unclear situation as rheumatism, of course the musculo-skeletal system must be aided, as must general body elimination. Beyond that it is difficult to be specific at this point as so many other parts of the body can be involved, depending upon the individual involved. For example:

- If it is the result of long standing sports injuries, then connective tissue must be strengthened, while using anti-spasmodics to ease the musculature.
- If the patient has a history of digestive problems, then the use of digestive tonics of the appropriate kind is indicated.
- Cardiovascular tonics should be used if there is any hypertension or even overt heart disease. The balance between herbs for active treatment of the rheumatism and the C-V problem rests upon the professional judgement of the herbalist.
- Long-term stress may lead to tense and tight muscles; this in turn may hold the joints too tightly thus resulting in friction. Over the years this will potentially develop into wear and tear osteo-arthritis, but in the short term it will cause pain and stiffness.

Specific remedies abound in the folk traditions for this common problem. Most of the salicylate-containing anti-inflammatories are considered specifics in the various folk traditions of the world. Especially important are Meadowsweet, Wintergreen, Quaking Aspen, Willow Bark. In addition we can add Angelica, Celery Seed and in fact all the anti-rheumatics mentioned above!

External applications will often help. These may be rubefacients, circulatory stimulants, salicin containing oils or even anti-spasmodics. It all depends upon what the patient responds best to.

From all that has been said it should be clear that a whole range of combinations might be appropriate for a specific individual. Here is one possible prescription:

> Willow Bark
> Meadowsweet
> Angelica
> Nettles

These herbs are combined in equal parts and then 1 teaspoonful (5 ml.) of tincture mixture is taken three times a day. If the dried herbs are being used then 2 teaspoonfuls of the combined herbs are infused to make one cup of herb tea. This should be drunk three or four times a day. In addition, benefit might be gained by using some sort of external application. This may be a stimulating liniment to increase local circulation and impart a sense of warmth, or a muscle relaxing anti-spasmodic rub.

The internal treatment provides a basic range of anti-rheumatics that give salicylate anti-inflammatory action along with support for the digestive process as well as a more generalised alterative. External treatments are so numerous that it is as much a matter of cultural preference as therapeutic judgement. Dietary factors must be considered (see below). A careful review of lifestyle will help clarify issues around posture, work conditions, stress, etc. Chiropractic, osteopathy, aromatherapy, massage and attention to appropriate exercise may prove most useful.

Osteo-arthritis
This is an all-too-common condition throughout the world, that is characterised by slow wearing down of the bony joints.

Again there are certain actions directly indicated for treating the process behind this disease:

- *Anti-rheumatics* will usually help but their selection must be based upon a sound therapeutic rationale.
- *Anti-inflammatories* are fundamental as their use will not only ease the symptom picture but help to stop the degenerative changes to bony tissue. In osteo-arthritis, the salicylate-based herbs are especially helpful.
- *Alteratives* are the key to any attempt at transforming the systemic problem (if present). If the osteo-arthritis has its roots in physical wear and tear they will not be quite so fundamental.
- *Anti-spasmodics* will lessen the impact of physical friction through relaxing the muscular envelope around the arthroses.
- *Circulatory stimulants* will benefit the healing process through increasing the flow-through of blood, thus facilitating all the work this amazing tissue fulfils.
- *Rubefacients* can be especially useful for local stimulation of circulation and inflammation reduction.
- *Analgesics* will possibly ease the patient's discomfort, but must not replace appropriate treatment.
- *Diuretics* help the kidney do its cleansing work.
- *Nervines* will usually be relevant because of the many ways in which a stressed patient can benefit from such support. The relaxants will also help as anti-spasmodics, the tonics will help the person deal with the constant stress of the pain and discomfort. Hypnotics will help them sleep in the face of pain.
- *Other actions* – such as bitters, hepatics, expectorants, emmenagogues. The whole digestive process must be working well and not damaged by side-effect reactions to non-steroidal anti-inflammatories.

Support for the rest of the body while it is dealing with the problems of osteo-arthritis is essential. In addition to musculo-skeletal attention, the digestive system needs special care. Beyond that it will depend upon the individual's specific case. Herbs to help good elimination of body waste are vital, without resorting to strenuous remedies that produce the 'purging and puking' so beloved by Victorian herbalists!

Again there are some impressive specific remedies available. Both Bogbean and Devil's Claw are usually considered to be specifics here. However, the multi-factorial roots of osteo-arthritis must be remembered, highlighting the unlikelihood of one totally specific remedy. Nettles are a traditional remedy throughout Europe, used internally and externally as a rubefacient. This external use, with fresh raw leaf, is not a treatment for the faint-hearted!

A possible prescription might look like this:

Bogbean	2 parts
Meadowsweet	1½ parts
Black Cohosh	1 part
Prickly Ash	1 part
Celery Seed	1 part
Angelica	1 part
Yarrow	1 part

Such a medicine would usually be made up as tinctures, as a tea would not be very pleasant! The dispensor would combine the herbs in the proportions mentioned and the patient would take up to 1 teaspoonful (5ml.) three times a day. This would be diluted in water and taken after food. If there is any associated stomach irritation due to the harshness of the Bogbean, then add Marshmallow Root. External treatments would be given as needed.

Why these herbs? Using the actions model described above, the prescription can be seen as offering a range of relevant actions supplied by combining different anti-rheumatics:

- *alterative remedies* – Bogbean and Black Cohosh
- *salicylate anti-inflammatories* – Meadowsweet
- *general anti-inflammatories* – Angelica, Bogbean and Black Cohosh
- *nervine anti-spasmodics* – Black Cohosh and Celery Seed
- *peripheral vasodilator* – Prickly Ash
- *diuretics* – Celery Seed and Yarrow

- 'stomachics', in this case *carminative* and intestinal anti-inflammatories – Angelica and Celery Seed
- *bitter tonics* – Bogbean and Yarrow

Nutritional factors are very important in the successful treatment of these problems, but there are many conflicting ideas about which foods or supplements to use for arthritis. While staying clear of such controversies, it is appropriate to focus on which foods to avoid as they definitely aggravate arthritic problems. A basic exclusion diet would include:

- coffee, whether decaf. or regular;
- red meat of any kind in any form;
- vinegar and anything based upon vinegar such as pickles; apple cider vinegar *may* possibly be an exception;
- vegetables that contain high levels of plant acids, e.g. tomatoes and rhubarb;
- berries rich in fruit acids such as Gooseberries, Red and Black Currants;
- refined white sugar and products that contain it;
- refined white flour and its multitude of products;
- artificial additives, flavourings and preservatives;
- processed foods;
- red wine, port and sherry;
- carbonated drinks;
- shell fish;
- any food or beverage that causes the patient specific problems.

Such diets will produce the best results in the earlier, more painful stages of this long-drawn-out disease. In the extreme of long standing osteo-arthritis, there is a balance that must be found between nutritional dogma that might not be too effective and eating habits that have a positive psychological effect on the patient.

Attention must be given to physical aids and support for the patient who is becoming disabled by this disease. There are a wealth of simple devices available that ease the simple daily tasks of life that have become taxing for the patient. These range from specially designed kitchen devices such as cutlery, tin-openers and tap-grips, to brushes with extended handles and adaptations to telephones. Using such aids can ease the patient's daily-life difficulties enormously.

THE NERVOUS SYSTEM

Perhaps the most dramatic and fascinating field of herbalism is the way in which plants affect consciousness. The integration revealed by the Gaia Hypothesis lays a philosophical foundation for this. Awareness and expanded consciousness are part of the life of the greater being of which we are part. Words and names are meaningless when considering such things, but just as our Earth feeds us, heals our arthritis and strengthens cardiac function, so the nervous system is supported and nurtured.

Herbalism is a co-operation between humanity, plants and the Earth in healing. This experience of wholeness is spirit in action, and opens the door for change, transformation and participation in the Great Work. Plants provide us with herbs that transform and enlighten, and also heal and nurture nerve tissue itself.

The whole therapy of herbalism is uniquely suited to treating nervous-system problems. From one perspective herbs are embodiments of energy and spirit, while from another they are packets of biochemicals. In fact a reflection of the human mind/brain itself! If used with awareness it is possible to address the needs of the human-energy body as well as the tissue involved. The complexities of the mind–body interface, that so confuse doctors concerned with 'psychosomatic' medicine, become an aid in remedy selection to the herbalist.

All of the many herbal nervines have impact on somatic symptoms as well as the mind. A simple example is Motherwort (*Leonurus cardiaca*), a herb used in treating anxiety and tension. It also has specific affinity for the heart, reducing palpitation reactions and the fear that often accompanies them. This is even recognised in the Latin binomial. This is discussed in depth in *Herbal Stress Control* by David Hoffmann and published by Thorsons.

Recent advances in the field of neurology have come about through the examination of claims for herbal remedies. Most of the areas of concern of neurology will potentially benefit from herbal therapeutics, and indeed the science of psycho-pharmacology itself is largely based on chemicals discovered in plants. Concerning therapy of nerve tissue as such, laboratory research, into the use of Ginkgo for a range of conditions which include Alzheimer's disease, Feverfew in the treatment of migraine and Siberian Ginseng for stress adaptation, are producing dramatic evidence of their efficacy.

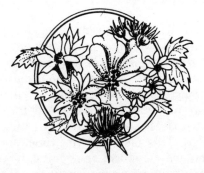

5 · PERSONAL HEALTH CARE WITH HERBS

Herbs are safe and effective remedies that make an ideal contribution as part of personal health-care programmes or of home medicine chests. As the knowledge and wisdom of the herbalist is the birthright of all people, it does not necessitate a professionally trained medical herbalist to use plant remedies for the minor ills that abound in family life, though for more serious problems the skills of a trained professional may be called for. The health and wholeness of ourselves and those we love is a vital concern, but one too often handed into someone else's care, and in these times of medical complexity and confusion, society has come to depend upon the expert. The benefits of our specialised health-care system have been paid for in many ways, one being a loss of personal responsibility for health and well-being, and although the skills of health-care workers are life-saving, society may have gone too far in empowering professional elites at the expense of self-help.

There is every reason to take care with personal health and wholeness, and herbalism makes a natural contribution.

But which remedies to choose and what conditions to treat? With the multitude of healing plants that are used in herbal medicine, what can be realistically provided in the home? An apparently daunting prospect faces the fledgling herbalist!

Selecting remedies to use and get to know is the first step. One way of doing this is to read through a herbal from A to Z (Abscess root to Zedoary!) until finding just what is needed. This takes a lot of time, and although it is an enjoyable way to spend an evening, it won't help the illness. Alternatively use a source book that lists conditions, describing herbal treatments. This is fine but limiting, as it means doing what the author tells you to do for a particular ailment, rather than taking into account that each sick person is unique and not simply a disease name. By applying the model used by the professional medical herbalist to the problem of which herbs to select for use in the home, a list of relevant, cheap and readily available herbs is quickly arrived at.

A HERBAL MEDICINE CHEST FOR THE HOME

It is a simple matter to stock a small herbal medicine chest which will fulfil most day-to-day needs. The following list of herbs includes representatives of all the important actions, but also commonly used specifics. Of course there are many alternatives, so if a favourite herb is not on the list, compare its actions and see what it would replace. On the other hand, simply switch herbs. If you are going to stock such a medicine chest, become thoroughly familiar with these plants, and use them at your discretion. They may be stored as tinctures, tablets or dried herbs. Dried herbs should be kept dry and airtight, away from direct light. Their specific uses are briefly described at the end of this chapter.

Boneset	Bogbean	Calendula (Marigold)
Chamomile	Cleavers	Dandelion
Echinacea	Feverfew	Ginkgo
Golden Seal	Hawthorn	Linden flower
Marshmallow	Meadowsweet	Milk Thistle
Mullein	Nettles	St John's Wort
Siberian Ginseng	Uva-Ursi	Valerian

In addition to these 'medicinal' herbs, there are the wonderful culinary herbs and spices that have valuable healing properties. Details on herbs such as Rosemary, Ginger, Mustard, Fennel and Aniseed will be found in all good herbals.

From the rich traditional roots of herbalism has come the knowledge of specific remedies for specific symptoms and diseases. This wealth of knowledge, based on generations of experience, provides the modern herbalist with a solid foundation from which to embrace the insights of science and contribute much to the new approaches of holistic medicine. However, for the person wanting to use herbs in their own health care, this abundance is overwhelming! The herbs that are discussed here can provide a whole spectrum of possibilities if their actions are compared and combined. This enables most common problems to be tackled by the novice herbalist, without necessitating an extensive home pharmacy. Most of the important actions are covered by the small number of herbs suggested here for the medicine chest.

Alterative: Cleavers, Dandelion, Echinacea, Garlic, Nettles

Anti-catarrhal: Boneset, Echinacea, Garlic, Golden Seal

Anti-inflammatory: Bogbean, Marigold, Chamomile, Feverfew, Meadowsweet, St John's Wort

Anti-microbial: Marigold, Chamomile, Echinacea, Elecampane, Garlic, Uva-Ursi

Anti-spasmodic: Boneset, Chamomile, Garlic, Linden Flowers, Valerian

Astringent: Golden Seal, Meadowsweet, Nettles, St John's Wort

Bitter: Bogbean, Chamomile, Dandelion, Feverfew, Golden Seal

Carminative: Chamomile, Meadowsweet, Linden Flowers, Valerian

Demulcent: Marshmallow, Milk Thistle, Mullein

Diaphoretic: Boneset, Elecampane, Garlic, Linden Flowers, Peppermint

Diuretic: Boneset, Cleavers, Dandelion, Linden Flowers, Meadowsweet, Mullein, Uva-Ursi

Emmenagogue: Marigold

Expectorant: Marshmallow, Mullein
Hepatic: Garlic, Dandelion, Golden Seal, Milk Thistle
Hypotensive: Garlic, Hawthorn, Linden Flowers, Valerian
Laxative: Boneset, Golden Seal,
Lymphatic: Marigold, Cleavers, Echinacea, Garlic
Nervine: Marigold, Chamomile, Linden Flowers, St John's Wort, Valerian
Tonic: Marigold, Chamomile, Cleavers, Echinacea, Garlic, Golden Seal, Hawthorn, Nettles
Vulnerary: Marigold, Marshmallow, Mullein, St John's Wort

Through applying the model of using a herbal action to address the physiological need of the individual, many health problems can be treated with this small number of remedies. Treatments for the following conditions will demonstrate the potentials for using this small number of remedies, but a more comprehensive herbal should be consulted for in-depth information or problems not discussed here.

MAINTAINING HEALTH AND PREVENTING ILLNESS

The old adage that prevention is better than cure is not only correct; with herbs it is easy to act on. A number of steps can be taken to nurture the health that even the most frail person is blessed with. This involves not only nurturing the body but caring for emotions and thoughts with the same depth of attention, for to be healthy we must be whole. Balance and harmony are the key to successful preventative medicine. There must be a clear and free flow of energy through the various aspects of the individual's life. Thus a range of issues must be addressed that go beyond the way herbal medicine can transform metabolic and physiological processes.

- *Nutrition* must be of a quality that enables the body to renew itself in a way that ensures health and wholeness.
- *Structural factors* must be addressed, by skilled practitioners if this is indicated, but also through appropriate exercise, dance or any enjoyable expression of bodily vitality.

- A conscious and free-flowing *emotional life* is fundamental to achieving any inner harmony.
- *Mental factors* are crucial: we are what we think!
- Openness to some form of *spirituality* is vital.

From these broad principle some ideas become clear that the herbalist can act upon. Most important in these times of ecocrisis and alienation from the natural world is to experience the embrace of nature, not only through using herbs but such things as walks in the woods or even hugging a tree. Smile!

Eat a healthy, balanced diet and ensure good bodily elimination, explored more below. Build any therapeutic programme undertaken around gentle tonic herbs, and not simply the strong remedies that focus on symptoms. Find a coping strategy for stress and the challenges of life that works for *you* and not simply the programme described in the lastest self-help best-seller. Remember that you are the only expert on you.

Use herbs to fortify any part of the body that needs support, as the plant kingdom is an abundant and rich resource for anyone interested in prevention. The key to prevention lies in an understanding of the role of herbal actions in maintaining health and appropriate physiological activity as herbs used in the right way will support the body's own process of maintaining a stable internal environment.

The concept of system tonics highlights the possibility of nourishing and toning the whole of a body system. This will aid both the structural form of the tissues and organs as well as functional activity, without eliciting a specific physiological or biochemical response. Bitter tonics as a group will have a generalised toning effect upon the body. The second herbal step is to use specific remedies or appropriate actions for any health problem that might be present. The third stage is to support normal functioning of eliminatory processes. Cleansing and detoxification can be gently facilitated through herbal support of the eliminatory systems of the body as described below.

ELIMINATION AND DETOXIFICATION

The human body is a miracle of beauty and efficiency, born with the ability to maintain health and wholeness. Much illness is the result of not supporting the body's own healing skills. Using herbal remedies that specifically aid and nurture the innate processes of healing and renewal, natural processes of body cleansing are supported. In the face of the pollutants around and within us, simply helping bodily detoxification and elimination goes a long way in the healing process. Using remedies for the specific problems, while supporting these eliminatory processes, speeds recovery from whatever illness is concerned.

Using simple and safe herbs will support this natural process, as long as the eliminative processes are addressed as a whole, and not just the colon, as is too often the case. This means that whenever such a programme is undertaken, ensure that all organs of elimination are being helped at the same time. In addition always help the specific area of the body that has been under most toxic pressure. Examples would be the lungs in a tobacco smoker or the liver in someone with alcohol-related problems. This process can be summarised as follows:

- Support the whole process of elimination.
- Specific support for overly taxed organs.
- Alleviate symptoms and address any pathologies that are also present.

The four primary pathways of elimination are the digestive system, kidneys, lungs and the skin. Each is vital and if one is not functioning well, the others carry an extra load. The digestive system cleanses via the colon and through the detoxification and natural laxative work of the liver. The use of strong herbal laxatives to empty the bowel should be avoided as they can lead to dependency. The best way to promote bowel cleansing is via the liver and the use of dietary fibre. The kidneys cleanse the blood and excrete waste via the urine. Herbal diuretics help this process. The skin eliminates waste via perspiration which is helped by diaphoretic remedies. Much more than carbon dioxide is eliminated via the lungs. Rub raw garlic on the soles of the feet and quite soon the distinctive aroma of garlic is on the breath! This is the body at work eliminating through the lungs. Herbal expectorants support this cleansing work. So to summarise the actions that help each body system:

- for the digestive system and colon – laxative
- for the liver and blood – hepatic, alterative
- for the kidneys and urinary system – diuretic
- for the lymphatic system – alterative, lymphatic tonic
- for the skin – diaphoretic, alterative
- for the respiratory system – expectorant, anti-catarrhal
- and for systemic support in general – tonic, alterative, adaptogen, anti-microbial

There are many plants that might be chosen. This diversity and abundance of healing plants is at once both the gift of herbalism and the frustration of the herb student! However there is a simple basic guideline to follow. Always use gentle remedies when stimulating elimination. If strong plants are used, the result may be overly dramatic. This is unpleasant, uncomfortable and of no therapeutic benefit.

Here are some suggestions for herbs that effectively supply the relevant actions while also being safe and mild. This is not a comprehensive list but examples taken from the medicine-chest list.

- laxative – Dandelion root
- diuretic – Dandelion Leaf, Cleavers, Uva-Ursi
- hepatic – Bogbean, Dandelion Root, Milk Thistle
- alterative – Nettles, Cleavers
- lymphatic tonic – Cleavers, Echinacea, Marigold
- diaphoretic – Boneset, Linden Flowers
- expectorant – Mullein
- tonic – any tonic remedy, described above, that has an affinity for the parts of the body under pressure from toxic build-up
- adaptogen – Siberian Ginseng
- anti-microbial – Echinacea, Garlic

INFECTIONS AND IMMUNITY

Human immunity has been stretched to the limits of its tolerance. In the face of pollution, food additives, chemical medicine, chemical food, it is no wonder that our resistance is suffering! The damage to the environment perpetrated in the name of 'progress' is damaging planetary health in a very similar way. The immune system has become an increasingly crucial issue in recent years. Not only in medicine but in many aspects of our lives, having a grasp of the new concepts concerning human immunity has become essential in understanding our world and making personal choices.

This is not only due to the AIDS epidemic but also the statistical explosion of a whole range of auto-immune diseases. To comprehend the possibilities of holistic approaches it is important to have a grasp of the biological basis of immunity, but at least as important is a comprehension of the role it plays in human life. The wonderful (yet partial) understanding that immunology grants us illuminates the great depth of complexity and ecological integration of the body, but there is much, much more involved. Herbal medicine is as limited as allopathic medicine if it is only used in a context of blood T- and B-cells without the benefit of a broader holistic context.

Some important insights arise when our immunity is placed in an ecological perspective and not simply a medical one. From such a perspective it becomes evident that human immunity is a vital component of the interface between the individual and their world. Human activity is not simply that of resisting the 'evil and dangerous' environment; rather it is a complex and beautiful dance of flowing to and fro within our world. Perceiving human immunity as a resistance process limits the possibilities for treatment. Of course resistance to disease is a fundamental component of the immune response, but not all of it. There is a constant dynamic interplay between the body and its world, and the immune system is part of a dialogue, an ecological dance between the within and the without of a human being. Rather than restricting therapy of the immune system to those things that build up resistance, we can introduce remedies that strengthen the ability to be open and receptive.

Ensuring a vibrant immune system involves taking care of the whole person. Through diet, exercise and safe medicine when needed, a healthy body will provide a firm foundation for immunity. Feelings too have a direct impact upon immune response, highlighting the need for emotional well-being.

Using the herbs suggested here will go a long way to support the body. A number of different levels can be supported herbally. For deep-seated immune support, there is fascinating new research on remedies from China that have a direct stimulating effect on immune-system response. Herbs such as Astragalus, the Shiitake mushroom and others have received much publicity. They are widely available, but need not be part of the medicine chest. The traditional tonic remedies of Western herbalism may well be providing similar immune support, but have attracted little research. Perhaps the Nettle is not glamorous enough! Nettles and Golden Seal from the list on p.100 may help as a tonic.

Nature provides a wealth of plants to support resistance to disease. Anti-microbial herbs such as Echinacea, Marigold, Golden Seal and Garlic can prevent and treat infection. In small amounts taken regularly they boost resistance, or larger doses combat specific infections. Diaphoretics such as Boneset, Linden flowers, Cayenne and Ginger also help.

Stress must be treated, as it has a direct impact on immunity. The more pressure endured, the more battering the immune system sustains. In addition to working with a stress-management programme, use adaptogenic herbs such as Siberian Ginseng.

HERBS FOR THE MEDICINE CHEST

In a book of this scope it is not possible to give the remedies the attention they deserve, but Chamomile, Valerian and Milk Thistle are considered in more depth elsewhere.

Boneset *Eupatorium perfoliatum*

Actions diaphoretic, aperient, anti-spasmodic, diuretic, anti-catarrhal, bitter

Boneset gets its name from the relief it gave for 'break bone fever' in the last century. It eases symptoms associated with influenza and other infections that feel 'fluish'. Although it does not directly combat the virus, it makes the whole experience more bearable by relieving the aches and pains. It may be used as symptomatic relief in muscular rheumatism. As a good diaphoretic it helps the body deal with any associated fever. It is effective in clearing sinus cattarh. Additionally its mild aperient (laxative), bitter and diuretic actions make Boneset a good general cleansing remedy.

Calendula (Marigold) *Calendula officinalis*

Actions Anti-inflammatory, astringent, vulnerary, anti-fungal, cholagogue, emmenagogue

A beautiful flower long used throughout Europe for wound-healing and ulcer treatments. Ideal for treating local skin problems, it may be used safely for inflammations on the skin, whether due to infection or to physical damage, and for any external bleeding or wound, bruising, strains, as well as in slow-healing wounds and skin ulcers. It is an ideal first-aid treatment of minor burns. Local treatments may be with a lotion, a poultice or compress. Internally it is used for digestive inflammations or ulceration. As a hepatic it aids treatment of gall-bladder problems and also through this can help in many of the vague digestive complaints that are called 'indigestion'. Marigold has anti-fungal activity and may be used both internally and externally to combat such infections. It is a normaliser of the menstrual process.

Cleavers *Galium aparine*

Actions Diuretic, alterative, anti-inflammatory, tonic, astringent, anti-neoplastic

Cleavers is a very valuable plant and possibly the best tonic for the lymphatic system available. As a lymphatic tonic with alterative and diuretic actions it may be used in a wide range of problems where the lymphatic system is involved. It is used in swollen glands anywhere in the body, especially for tonsillitis and adenoids. Widely used in skin conditions, Cleavers specifically treats dry conditions such as psoriasis. It is used for the treatment of cystitis and other urinary conditions. There is a long tradition for the use of Cleavers in the treatment of ulcers and tumours, which may be the result of the lymphatic drainage.

Coltsfoot   *Tussilago farfara*

Actions Expectorant, anti-tussive, demulcent, anti-catarrhal, diuretic

Coltsfoot combines a soothing expectorant effect with an anti-spasmodic action. There are useful levels of zinc in the leaves. This mineral has been shown to be anti-inflammatory. Coltsfoot is used in chronic or acute bronchitis, irritating coughs, whooping coughs and asthma. Its soothing expectorant action gives Coltsfoot a role in most respiratory conditions, including emphysema. As a mild diuretic it has been used in cystitis. The fresh bruised leaves can be applied to boils, abscesses and suppurating ulcers.

Echinacea   *Echinacea augustifolia*

Actions anti-microbial, alterative

Echinacea is the prime remedy to help the body rid itself of microbial infections. Immunity is helped via a stimulation of white blood corpuscle production and a polysaccharide that is anti-viral. Effective against both bacterial and viral attacks, it may be used in conjunction with other herbs for infection anywhere in the body. For example in combination with Uva-Ursi it effectively treats cystitis. Especially useful for infections of the upper respiratory tract such as laryngitis, tonsillitis, and for catarrhal conditions of the nose and sinus. As a mouthwash it speeds the treatment of pyorrhoea and gingivitis. It may be used as an external lotion to help septic sores and cuts.

Golden Seal   *Hydrastis canadensis*

Actions tonic, astringent, anti-catarrhal, anti-microbial, laxative, oxytocic, bitter

One of our most useful remedies owing much of its value to the tonic effects it has on the mucous membranes of the body. This is why it is of such help in all digestive problems, from peptic ulcers to colitis. Its bitter stimulation helps in loss of appetite, and the alkaloids it contains stimulate bile production and secretion. All catarrhal conditions improve with Golden Seal, especially sinus ones. The anti-microbial properties appear to be due to alkaloids present. Traditionally it has been used during labour to help contractions, but it is for just this reason that it should be avoided during pregnancy. Applied externally it can be helpful in eczema, ringworm, itching, earache and conjunctivitis.

Marshmallow   *Althaea officinalis*

Actions   root: demulcent, diuretic, emollient, vulnerary
Leaf: demulcent, expectorant, diuretic, emollient
The high mucilage content of Marshmallow makes it an excellent demulcent that can be used wherever needed. The root is used primarily for digestive problems and on the skin; the leaf for the lungs and the urinary system. In all inflammations of the digestive tract, such as those of the mouth, gastritis, peptic ulcer, enteritis and colitis, the root is best. For bronchitis, respiratory catarrh and irritating coughs the leaves should be considered. It is also soothing in cases of urethritis and urinary gravel. In fact it soothes mucous membrane anywhere. Externally, the root is used in varicose veins and ulcers as well as abscesses and boils.

Peppermint   *Mentha piperita*

Actions   carminative, anti-spasmodic, aromatic, diaphoretic, anti-emetic, nervine, antiseptic, analgesic
Peppermint is an excellent carminative, having a relaxing effect on the muscles of the digestive system, combats flatulence and stimulates bile and digestive juice flow. It is used to relieve intestinal colic, flatulent dyspepsia and associated conditions. The volatile oil acts as a mild anaesthetic to the stomach wall, which allays feelings of nausea and the desire to vomit. It helps to relieve the nausea and vomiting of pregnancy and travel sickness. Peppermint

can play a role in the treatment of ulcerative conditions of the bowels. It is a traditional treatment for fevers, colds and influenza. As an inhalant it is used as temporary relief for nasal catarrh. Where headaches are associated with digestion, Peppermint may help. As a nervine it eases anxiety and tension. In painful periods, it relieves the pain and eases associated tension. Externally it is used to relieve itching and inflammations.

Uva-Ursi   *Arctostaphylos uva-ursi*

Actions   Diuretic, anti-microbial, astringent

An effective treatment for cystitis, this oil-rich leaf may be used in any infection of the urinary system. It will soothe associated inflammation in the bladder and other areas. Will help in the treatment of kidney stones and gravel. Uva-Ursi makes a good general diuretic.

HEALING REMEDIES FROM THE KITCHEN

Food is the best medicine, for it is from our nutrition that we nurture the life in us. Herbal remedies are simply a specific variety of vegetables and a vital part of nature's garden. Here we shall consider some of the healing potential of the herbs and spices found in most kitchens. There is not the space to consider the fruits and vegetables – that is a whole other book!

Marjoram   *Origanum vulgare*

Actions   stimulant, diaphoretic, antiseptic, expectorant, emmenagogue, rubefacient

Marjoram is a widely used herb in folk remedies and cooking. As a stimulating diaphoretic it is often used in the treatment of colds and 'flu. Its mild antiseptic properties help when used as a mouthwash for inflammations of the mouth and throat. The infusion is used in coughs and whooping cough. Headaches, expecially when due to tension, may be relieved by a tea of Marjoram or by rubbing the forehead and temples with the oil. The oil may also be used for rubbing into areas of muscular and rheumatic pain. A lotion will soothe stings and bites and be antiseptic for infected cuts and wounds.

Rosemary *Rosmarinus officinalis*

Actions carminative, aromatic, anti-spasmodic, anti-depressive, antiseptic, rubefacient, parasiticide

Rosemary is a circulatory and nervine stimulant, which in addition to the toning and calming effect on the digestion is used where psychological tension is present. This may show for instance as flatulent dyspepsia, headache or depression associated with debility. Externally it may be used to ease muscular pain, sciatica and neuralgia. It acts as a stimulant to the hair follicles and may be used in premature baldness. The oil is most effective here.

Fennel *Foeniculum vulgare*

Actions carminative, aromatic, anti-spasmodic, stimulant, galactogogue, rubefacient, expectorant

Fennel is an excellent stomach and intestinal remedy which relieves flatulence and colic while also stimulating the digestion and appetite. It is similar to Aniseed in its calming effect on bronchitis and coughs and is used to flavour cough remedies. Fennel will increase the flow of milk in nursing mothers. Externally the oil eases muscular and rheumatic pains. The infusion may be used to treat conjunctivitis and inflammation of the eyelids as a compress.

Dill *Anethum graveolens*

Actions carminative, aromatic, anti-spasmodic, galactogogue

Dill is an excellent remedy for flatulence and the colic that is sometimes associated with it. This is the herb of choice in the colic of children. It will stimulate the flow of milk in nursing mothers. Chewing the seeds will help clear bad breath.

Cayenne *Capsicum minimum*

Actions stimulant, carminative, tonic, sialagogue, rubefacient, antiseptic

Cayenne is the most useful of the systemic stimulants. It stimulates blood flow, strengthening the heart, arteries, capillaries and nerves. A general tonic it is also specific for the circulatory and digestive system. It may be used in flatulent dyspepsia and colic. If there is insufficient peripheral circulation, leading to cold hands and feet and possibly chilblains, Cayenne may be used; also for debility and for warding off colds. Externally it is used as a rubefacient in problems like lumbago and rheumatic pains. As an ointment it helps unbroken chilblains, as long as it is used in moderation! As a gargle in laryngitis it combines well with Myrrh. This combination is also a good antiseptic wash.

Aniseed   *Pimpinella anisum*

Actions   expectorant, anti-spasmodic, carminative, parasiticide, aromatic

The volatile oil in Aniseed provides the basis for its internal use in easing griping, intestinal colic and flatulence. It also has a marked expectorant and anti-spasmodic action and may be used in bronchitis, in tracheitis where there is persistent irritable coughing, and in whooping cough. Externally, the oil may be used in an ointment base for the treatment of scabies. The oil by itself will help in the control of lice.

Celery Seeds   *Apium graveolens*

Actions   anti-rheumatic, diuretic, carminative, sedative

Celery Seeds find their main medical use in the treatment of rheumatism, arthritis and gout. They are especially useful in rheumatoid arthritis where there is an associated mental depression. Their diuretic action is obviously involved in rheumatic conditions, but they are also used as a urinary antiseptic, largely because of the volatile oil apiol.

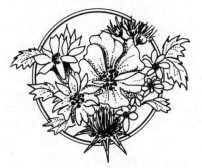

6 · PREPARING HERBS SO THAT THEY WORK!

Herbalism is rich in medicine-making techniques. Our ancestors probably ate the plants fresh. In the many years of herbal history that followed those early wildcrafters, other methods of preparing remedies have been developed, enabling their healing properties to be released and activated. Marrying the legacy of generations of herbalists with understanding a modicum of pharmacology makes informed choices about techniques and processes easy. Practical details can be found in all modern comprehensive herbals.

A method of preparation must be selected which releases the biochemical constituents needed for healing without insulting the integrity of the plant by isolating fractions of the whole. The property of any herb is not simply the sum of the various chemicals present, as there is a synergy at work that creates a therapeutic whole that is more than the sum of its parts. If the method of preparation destroys or loses part of the whole, much of the healing power is lost.

Herbal teas, or tisanes, are the easiest way of preparing the remedies. There are some basic rules of thumb for choosing which method to use with what herb, but as with all generalisations, there are many exceptions! A simple example is that infusions are appropriate for non-woody material such as leaves, flowers and some stems, while decoctions are necessary if the herb contains any hard or woody material such as roots, barks or nuts. The denser the plant or the individual cell walls, the more energy is needed to extract cell content into the tea, which explains the value of decocting. An important exception would be a root rich in a volatile oil such as Valerian, for although the woodyness would suggest decocting, if simmered the therapeutically important volatile oil would boil off.

INFUSIONS

If you can make a cup of tea, you can make an infusion. As the simplest method of preparing a herb tea, both fresh or dried herbs may be used. Where one part of dried herb is prescribed, it can be replaced with three parts of the fresh herb, the difference being due to the higher water content of the fresh herb. To make an infusion:

- Put about 1 teaspoonful of the dried herb or herb mixture into a teapot for each cup.
- Add boiling water and cover. Leave to steep for 10–15 minutes. Infusions may be drunk hot, cold, or have ice in them. They may be sweetened.

Infusions are most appropriate for plant parts such as leaves, flowers or green stems where the substances wanted are easily accessible. To infuse bark, root, seeds or resin, it is best to powder them first to break down some of their cell walls and make them more accessible to the water. Seeds like Fennel and Aniseed should be slightly bruised to release the volatile oils from the cells. Any aromatic herb should be infused in a pot that has a well-sealing lid, to reduce loss of volatile oil through evaporation.

DECOCTIONS

For hard and woody herbs it is best to make a decoction rather than an infusion, ensuring that the soluble contents of the herb actually reach the water. Roots, rhizomes, wood, bark, nuts and some seeds are hard and their cell walls are very strong, so more heat is needed than for infusions and the herb has to be boiled in the water. To make a decoction:

- Put 1 teaspoonful of dried herb or 3 teaspoonfuls of fresh material for each cup of water into a pot or saucepan. Dried herbs should be powdered or broken into small pieces, while fresh material should be cut into small pieces.
- Add the appropriate amount of water to the herbs.
- Bring to the boil and simmer for 10–15 minutes.

When using a woody herb that contains a lot of volatile oils, it is best to make sure that it is powdered as finely as possible and then used in an infusion, to ensure that the oils do not boil away. Decoctions can be used in the same way as an infusion.

TINCTURES

Alcohol is a better solvent than water for the plant constituents. Mixtures of alcohol and water dissolve nearly all the ingredients of a herb and at the same time act as a preservative. Alcohol preparations are called tinctures.

When tinctures are prepared professionally according to descriptions in a pharmacopoeia, specific water/alcohol proportions are used for each herb, but for general use such details are unnecessary. For home use it is best to take an alcohol of at least 30 per cent (60 proof), vodka for instance, as this is about the weakest alcohol/water mixture with a long-term preservative action. To make an alcoholic tincture:

- Put 120 gm (4 oz) cut dried herb into a container that can be tightly closed. If fresh herbs are used, twice the amount should be taken.
- Pour half a litre (1 pint) of 30 per cent (60 proof) vodka on the herbs and close tightly.
- Keep the container in a warm place for two weeks, shaking once a day.
- After decanting the bulk of the liquid, pour the residue into a muslin cloth suspended in a bowl.

- Wring out all the liquid. The residue makes excellent compost.
- Pour the tincture into a well-stoppered dark bottle.

As tinctures are much stronger, volume for volume, than infusions or decoctions, the dosage to be taken is much smaller. They can be taken straight or mixed with a little water, or they can be added to a cup of hot water. If this is done, the alcohol will partly evaporate and leave most of the extract in the water, which with some herbs will make the water cloudy, as resins and other constituents not soluble in water will precipitate. Some drops of the tincture can be added to a bath or footbath, or used in a compressor mixed with oil and fat to make an ointment. Suppositories and lozenges can be made this way too.

VINEGAR-BASED TINCTURES

Tinctures can also be made using vinegar, which contains acetic acid that acts a solvent and preservative in a way similar to alcohol. Whenever you make a vinegar tincture, it is best to use apple cider vinegar, as it has in itself excellent health-augmenting properties. Synthetic chemical vinegar should not be used. The method is the same as for alcoholic tinctures and if you steep spices or aromatic herbs in vinegar, the resulting fragrant vinegar will be excellent for culinary use.

GLYCERINE-BASED TINCTURES

Tinctures based on glycerine have the advantage of being milder on the digestive tract than alcoholic tinctures, but they have the disadvantage of not dissolving resinous or oily materials quite as well. As a solvent, glycerine is generally better than water but not as good as alcohol.

To make a glycerine tincture, make up half a litre (1 pint) of a mixture consisting of one-part glycerine and one-part water, add 110 gm (4 oz) of the dried ground herb and leave it in a well-stoppered container for two weeks, shaking it daily. After two weeks, strain and press or wring the residue as with alcoholic tinctures. For fresh herbs, due to their greater water content, put 220 gm (8 oz) into a mixture of 75 per cent glycerine/25 per cent water.

SYRUPS

In the case of fluid medicine – be it infusion, decoction or tincture – that has a particularly unpleasant taste, it is sometimes advisable to mask the taste by combining the fluid with a sweetener. One way to do this is to use a syrup, which is the traditional way to make cough mixtures more palatable for children, or any herbal preparation more 'toothsome', as Culpeper used to call it.

A simple syrup base is made as follows: pour half a litre (1 pint) of boiling water on to 1.1 kg (2½ lb) of sugar, place over heat and stir until the sugar dissolves and the liquid begins to boil. Then take off the heat immediately. This simple syrup can best be used together with a tincture: mix one part of the tincture with three parts of syrup and store for future use. For use with an infusion or decoction, it is simpler to add the sugar directly to the liquid: for every half litre (one pint) of liquid add 350 gm (¾ lb) of sugar and heat gently until the sugar is dissolved. This again can be stored for future use and will keep quite well in a refrigerator. Since too much sugar is not very healthy, syrups are best used for gargles and cough medicines only.

CAPSULES AND PILLS

Using herbs in a dry form has the advantage that you can take the whole herb, including the woody material. The main drawback lies in the fact that the dry herbs are unprocessed, and so some constituents may not be readily absorbable. In a process like infusion, heat and water help to break down the walls of the plant cells and to dissolve the constituents, something which is not always guaranteed during the digestive process in the stomach and the small intestines. Also, when the constituents are already dissolved in liquid form, they are available a lot faster and begin their action sooner. Another drawback lies in the fact that, if taken as capsules, you do not taste the herb. For various reasons – even though they taste unpleasant – the bitter herbs work much better when they are tasted, as their effectiveness depends on the neurological sensation of bitterness. When you put bitters into a capsule or a pill, their action may well be lost or diminished.

The easiest way to use dry powdered herbs internally is to use gelatine capsules. The size needed depends on the amount of herbs prescribed per dose and on the volume of the material. A capsule size '00' for instance will hold about 0.5 gm ($\frac{1}{8}$ oz) of finely powdered herb. To fill a capsule is very easy:

- Place the powdered herbs in a flat dish and take the halves of the capsules apart.
- Move the halves of the capsules through the powder, filling them in the process.
- Push the halves together.

As the body can absorb herbal compounds through the skin, a wide range of methods and formulations have been developed that take advantage of this fact. Douches and suppositories, though they might appear to be internal remedies, have traditionally been categorised as external remedies.

BATHS

A very pleasant way of absorbing herbs through the skin is by having a bath with half a litre (1 pint) of infusion or decoction added to the water. For a foot- or hand-bath use the preparations in undiluted form. Any herb that can be taken internally may be used in a bath and, if chosen wisely, will add an excellent fragrance. Aromatherapy, a healing system based on the use of herbs in the form of essential oils, utilises baths by putting a few drops of the relevant oil into the water. Instead of preparing an infusion of the herb beforehand, a handful of it can also be placed in a muslin bag which is suspended from the hot-water tap so that the water flows through it. In this way a very fresh infusion can be made.

DOUCHES

This is a method particularly indicated for local infections. Whenever possible, prepare a new infusion or decoction for each douche. Allow the tea to cool to a temperature that will be comfortable internally. Pour it into the container of a douche bag and insert the applicator vaginally. Allow the liquid to rinse the inside of the vagina. Note that the liquid will run out of the vagina, so it is easiest to douche sitting on the toilet. It is not necessary to actively hold in the liquid. In most conditions indicating a need for douching, it is advisable to use the tea undiluted for a number of days three times daily. If, however, a 3–7 day course of douching (along with the appropriate internal herb remedies) has not noticeably improved a vaginal infection, see a qualified practitioner for a diagnosis.

OINTMENTS

Ointments or salves are semi-solid preparations that can be applied to the skin. Depending on the purpose for which they are designed, there are innumerable ways of making ointments; they can vary in texture from very greasy ones to those made into a thick paste, depending on what base is used and on what compounds are mixed together.

Any herb can be used for making ointments, but Arnica Flower, Chickweed, Comfrey Root, Cucumber, Elder Flower, Eucalyptus, Golden Seal, Lady's Mantle, Marigold Flower, Marshmallow Root, Plantain, Slippery Elm Bark, Yarrow and Woundwort are particularly good for use in external healing mixtures.

The simplest way to prepare an ointment is by using Vaseline or a similar petroleum jelly as a base. Although this has the disadvantage of being an inorganic base, it also has a number of advantages. Vaseline is easy to handle, so a simple ointment can be made very quickly. The basic method for a Vaseline ointment is to simmer 2 tablespoonfuls of a herb in 200 gm (7 oz) of Vaseline for about 10 minutes. A single herb, a mixture, fresh or dried herbs, roots, leaves or flowers can be used.

Here is a recipe for a simple Marigold ointment, excellent for cuts, sores and minor burns:

- Take 60 gm (2 oz or about a handful) of freshly picked Marigold Flowers and 200 gm (7 oz) of Vaseline.

- Melt the Vaseline over low heat, add the Marigold Flowers and bring the mixture to the boil.
- Simmer it very gently for about 10 minutes, stirring well.
- Sift through fine gauze and press out all the liquid from the flowers.
- Pour the liquid into a container and seal it after it has cooled.

For vegetable based alternatives use beeswax and olive oil.

SUPPOSITORIES

Suppositories are designed to enable the insertion of remedies into the orifices of the body. They act as carriers for appropriate herbs. There are herbs that soothe mucous membranes, reducing inflammations and aid the healing process, such as Comfrey, Marshmallow, Golden Seal and Slippery Elm. There are also astringent herbs that reduce discharges, such as Periwinkle and Pilewort. It will often be appropriate to include anti-microbial herbs.

As with ointments, we can choose from different bases, keeping in mind that the suppository has to be firm enough for insertion and, at the same time being able to melt at body temperature once inserted. To prepare a simple suppository, mix the finely powdered herb with melted cocoa butter. Prepare a mould from aluminium foil which has been shaped appropriately. The best shape is a torpedo-like, 1-inch-long suppository. Pour the molten base into the mould and let it cool. Store in a refrigerator untill needed. To avoid the introduction of powdered plant material into the body, a more complex method has to be used, as described in more comprehensive books on herbs.

OILS

Pure essential oils, extracted from the herb by a complex and careful process of distillation, are best obtained from specialist suppliers. If purity is not an issue, a simple method of extracting oils infuses the herb in an oil, so obtaining a solution of the plant oil in the oil-base. Base oils to use are vegetable oils such as Olive, Sunflower, or Almond oil, but any good pressed vegetable oil can be used and these are preferable to mineral oils.

To make a herbal oil, first cut the herb finely, cover it with oil and put in a clear glass container. Place this in the sun or leave in a warm place for two or three weeks, shaking the container daily. After that time, filter the liquid into a dark glass container and store the extracted oil. St John's Wort makes a beautiful red oil that is used externally for massage and to help sunburns and heal wounds. To make it, pick the flowers when they are just opened and crush them in 1 teaspoonful of olive oil. Cover them with more oil, mix well and put in a glass container in the sun or a warm place for three to six weeks, at the end of which the oil will be bright red. Press the mixture through a cloth to remove all the oil and leave it to stand for a while, as there will be some water in the liquid which will settle on the bottom so that the oil can be decanted. Then store the oil in a well-sealed, dark container.

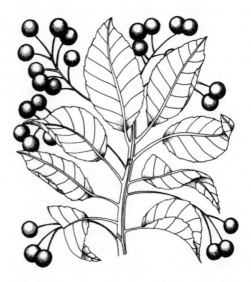

Figure 5   *Barberry*

COMPRESSES

This an excellent way of applying a remedy to the skin. Soak a clean linen or cotton cloth in a hot herbal tea and apply it to the affected part of the body. Use as hot as can be tolerated, and cover with a towel to hold in the heat. When cool replace with another. For a cold compress use the same method but simply let the tea cool.

POULTICES

This more therapeutically active method uses fresh or dried plants rather than a liquid form. Mash or crush fresh plant material and either heat over boiling water or mix with a small amount of boiling water to make a paste. Apply directly to the skin as hot as possible, and hold it in place with gauze. Powder dried herb and mix with hot water to create a paste. If using stimulating herbs such as Mustard, apply them between two layers of cloth.

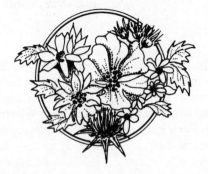

HERBAL NEXT STEPS

If this book has whetted your appetite and you would like to explore herbalism further, here are some suggestions.

- Visit nature. Spend time in natural wild places, and experience yourself as being truly part of our world.
- Get to know the herbs. Learn to identify them, know where they live and grow.
- Grow the herbs. This may be in a garden or in little pots.
- Use them for health care and as an enhancement of life. Make cosmetics, flower wreaths, cook with them, etc. You will be surprised at the ways in which herbs can be part of your life.
- Further your education in herbalism.

HERBAL CONTACTS IN BRITAIN

The venerable herbal tradition in Britain is maintained and furthered today by the world's foremost professional body of herbal practitioners, the National Institute of Medical Herbalists. The public can be assured that members of this organisation are competent, ethical, professional medical practitioners. For more information about the institute and a members' list, please contact:

The National Institute of Medical Herbalists
41 Hatherley Road
Winchester
Hants SO22 6RR

With such a long tradition of high-quality herbal medicine, it is not surprising that one of the world's best schools for the professional training of medical herbalists is to be found in Britain. They offer a range of different courses depending upon the student's needs and educational level. Successful graduation entitles the student to join the National Institute of Medical Herbalists. The address is:

The School of Herbal Medicine PhytoTherapy
Bucksteep Manor
Bodle Street Green
Hailsham BN27 4RJ

A number of other schools have been started. They offer an education that reflects differences of philosophy and therapeutic approach. Study with these schools does not lead to membership of the Institute.

Dr Christopher's School of Natural Healing
19 Park Terrace
Stroke on Trent
Staffs

School of Natural Medicine
Dolphin House
6 Gold Street
Saffron Walden
Essex CB10 1EJ

The General Council & Register of Consultant Herbalists Ltd.
Malborough House
Swanpool
Falmouth
Cornwall TR11 4HW

The School of Chinese Herbal Medicine
Pine Trees
Chiltern Road
Amersham
Bucks HP6 5PG

Many organisations are involved with bringing herbalism to the public or to the attention of government bodies. The National Institute of Medical Herbalists is both helpful and important in its work. Other groups include:

The British Herbal Medicine Association
The Old Coach House
Southborough Road
Surbiton
Surrey

The Register of Chinese Herbal Medicine
7a Stanhope Road
London N6 5NE

The British Herb Grower's Association
17 Hooker Street
London SW3

The Herb Society
77 Great Peter Street
London SW1P 2EZ

HERBAL CONTACTS IN THE USA

Herbalism in the USA is in the paradoxical position of experiencing a flowering of interest in all its aspects, yet having few educational avenues to explore. This is one of the very few developed countries where medical herbalism is not legally recognised, making professional training a challenge! A move to change this anachronistic state of affairs has started with the launching of the American Herbalists Guild. For more information contact:

The American Herbalists Guild
PO Box 1127
Forestville
California 95436

As there is no licensing body, no degree-giving schools of herbalism currently exist. Naturopathic medicine covers the basics within the context of its broad approach, as do the acupuncture colleges for oriental herbalism. The National College of Naturopathic Medicine in Portland, Oregon and John Bastyr College in Seattle, Washington have good 'botanic' medicine courses.

The best herbal education is offered by schools that are educationally unorthodox. Such places have developed where herbalists live, rather than where the demand is. They are small-scale and on the whole excellent. As they are expressions of the vision, skills and wisdom of the herbalists involved, they have their unique strengths and weaknesses. Some offer full-time training, others are based on workshop formats or correspondence courses. For a comprehensive listing of such schools contact:

California School of Herbal Studies
PO Box 39
Forestville,
California 95436

Other useful addresses include:

The American Herb Association (publishers of an excellent newsletter)
Box 353
Rescue
California 96672

Herbalgram (another excellent journal)
PO Box 12602
Austin
Texas 78711

HERBAL CONTACTS IN CANADA

The Ontario Herbalists Association
181 Brookdale Avenue
Toronto
Ontario, M5M 1P4

HERBAL CONTACTS IN NEW ZEALAND

The New Zealand College of Naturopathic Medicine
Christchurch
New Zealand

HERBAL CONTACTS IN AUSTRALIA

The National Herbalists Association of Australia
49 Oakwood Street
Sutherland
New South Wales 2232

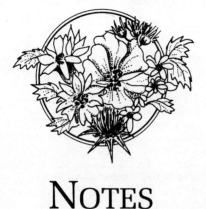

NOTES

1. J. Lovelock, *GAIA: A New Look at Life on Earth*, (Oxford University Press, 1979).
2. *WHO Technical Report* 622 (1978), The promotion and development of traditional medicine.
3. Leathwood *et al.*, Aqueous extract of valerian root (*Valeriana officinalis* L.) improves sleep quality in man, *Pharmacol. Biochem. Behav.* (1982 Jul.) 17(1); 65–71.
4. Balderer and Borbely, Effect of Valerian on human sleep, *Psychopharmacology* (1985) 87(4); 406–9.
5. Muller-Limmroth and Ehrenstein; Experimental studies of the effects of Seda-Kneipp on the sleep of sleep disturbed subjects; implications for the treatment of different sleep disturbances, *Med-Klin.* (1977 Jun. 24) 72(25); 1119–25.
6. Hazelhoff *et al.*, Anti-spasmodic effects of valeriana compounds, *Arch. Int. Pharmacodyn. Ther.* (1982 Jun.) 257(2); 274–87.
7. P.J. Houghton, The biological activity of Valerian and related plants; *J. Ethnopharmacol* (1988 Feb.–Mar.) 22(2); 121–42.
8. Dunaev *et al.*, Biological activity of the sum of the valepotriates isolated from *Valeriana alliariifolia*, *Farmakol Toksikol* (1987 Nov.–Dec.) 50(6); 33–7.
9. Della Loggia *et al.*, Evaluation of the activity on the mouse CNS of several plant extracts and a combination of them, *Riv. Neurol.* (1981 Sep.–Oct.) 51(5); 297–310.
10. J.R. Hanson, Diterpenoids. In Overton (ed.), *Terpenoids and Steroids* (London: The Chemistry Soc. 1974) pp.145–70.
11. Iatsyno *et al.*, Pharmacology of calenduloside B, a new triterpene glycoside from the roots of *Calendula officinalis*, *Farmakol Toksikol* (1978 Sep.–Oct.) 41(5); 556–60.
12. Levine, The Mexican plant zoapatle (*Montanoa tomentosa*) in reproductive medicine. Past, present and future, *J. Reprod. Med.* (1981 Oct.)

26(10); 524–8.

13. A.J. Gallegos et al., The zoapatle I – a traditional remedy from Mexico emerges to modern times, Contraception (1983 Mar.) 27(3); 211–25.

14. L. Southam et al., The zoapatle IV – toxicological and clinical studies, Contraception (1983 Mar.) 27(3); 255–65.

15. Hahn et al., Antifertility activity of Montanoa tomentosa, Contraception (1981 Feb.) 23(2); 133–40.

16. H. Ponce-Monter et al., The zoapatle X. The in vitro effect of zoapatle aqueous crude extract (ZACE) and histamine upon rat and guinea pig uterine strips, Contraception (1985 May) 31(5); 533–41.

17. Kong et al., Fertility regulating agents from traditional Chinese medicines, J. Ethnopharmacol. (1986 Jan.) 15(1); 1–44.

18. Kholkute and Udupa, Effects of Hibiscus rosa sinensis on fertility of rats, Planta Medica (1976) Vol. 29, 321–9.

19. J.L. Hartwell, Plants used against cancer. A survey. Lloydia 30 (1967), 379–436.

20. J.L. Hartwell, Plants used against cancer. A survey. Lloydia 32 (1971), 204–55.

21. Cassady and Douros, Anticancer Agents Based on Natural Product Models (New York: Academic Press, 1980).

22. G.A. Cordell, Anticancer agents from plants., Progr. Phytochem., 5, 273.

23. Gottlieb et al., Cancer Chemother. Res., 54 (1970), 461.

24. S. Mills, Dictionary of Modern Herbalism (Thorsons, 1986).

25. Beaune, Anti-inflammatory experimental properties of marshmallow: its potentiating action on the local effects of corticoids, Therapie (1966 Mar.–Apr.) 21(2); 341–7.

26. H. Glatzel, Effect of bitters on cardiac output, heart rate and blood pressure, Planta Med. (1968 Feb.) 16(1); 82–94.

27. Bhattacharya et al., Chemical constituents of gentianaceae XI. Antipsychotic activity of gentianine, J. Pharm. Sci. (1974 Aug.) 63(8); 134–2.

28. British Herbal Pharmacopoea (BHMA, 1983).

29. Glowania et al., Effect of chamomile on wound healing – a clinical double-blind study, Z Hautkr (1987 Sep. 1) 62(17); 1262, 1267–71.

30. Szelenyi, Pharmacological experiments with compounds of chamomile. III. Experimental studies of the ulcerprotective effect of chamomile, Planta Med. (1979 Mar.) 35(3); 218–27.

31. Vilagines, Delaveau and Vilagines, Inhibition of poliovirus replication by an extract of Matricaria chamomilla (L) C.R. Acad. Sci. [III] (1985) 301(6); 289–94.

32. Grabarczyk et al., Sesquiterpene lactones. Part XV. New cytostatic active sesquiterpene lactone from herb of Anthemis nobilis L. Pol. J. Pharmacol. Pharm. (1977 Jul.–Aug.) 29(4); 419–23.

33. F. Roberts, The Encyclopedia of Digestive Disorders, Thorsons.

34. G. Lavrenova and I.P. Chernov, Comparative evaluation of the effect of plant polysaccharides on the inflammatory process and regeneration in chronic stomach ulcer, Farmakol. Toksikol. (1983 Jul.–Aug.) 46(4); 85–9.

35. Baumann, Clinico-experimental studies on the secretion of bile, pancreatic and gastric juice under the influence of phytocholagogous agents of a suspension of *Carduus marianus, Chelidonium* and *Curcuma, Arzneim Forsch* (1971 Jan.) 21(1), 98–101.

36. Hahn *et al.*, On the pharmacology and toxicology of silymarin, an antihepatotoxic active principle from *Silybum marianum* (L.), *Arzneim Forsch* (1968 Jun.) 18(6), 698–704.

37. Fiebig, New antihepatotoxic effects of flavonolignans of a white flowering variety of *Silybum, Planta Med.* (1984 Aug.) 50(4); 310–13.

38. Vogel *et al.*, Proceedings: Neutralization of the lethal effects of phalloidine and alpha-amanitine in animal experiments by substances from the seeds of *Silybum marianum* l. gaertn., *Naunyn Schmiedebergs Arch. Pharmacol.* (1974 22 Mar.) 282(0); suppl. 282:R102.

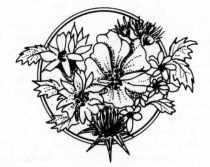

BIBLIOGRAPHY

There is a bewildering array of books about herbs, their uses, cultivation, preparation and their folk lore. There is also an ever-growing number of wonderful books pointing us in the direction of rapport with Gaia and of being truly present in our world.

Any suggested reading list offered here can be at best only small and partial, but some guidelines may prove useful. When considering a herbal new to you, consider these points:

- Is the author experienced in the area he or she is writing about? All too often the plethora of new herbals assailing the public are written by journalists commissioned by publishers to fill their subject catalogues. Although they usually write better than herbalists, the subject matter will usually come from other books.
- Read what the author has to say about a herb you know. Does he or she say anything new? Is this new information correct? If it is the same material but written about in a clear way, this may be very useful, as herbalists tend not to be the best writers! If there are actual mistakes then avoid that book.
- Read what the author has to say about the herbal treatment of an illness you know about. Is his or her approach one that adds insight to that of other authors you might already use?

British Herbal Pharmacopoeia (British Herbal Medicine Association, 1979).
Christopher, Dr John R., *School of Natural Healing* (BiWorld, 1976).
Gosling, Nalda, *Successful Herbal Remedies* (Thorsons, 1985).
Grieve, Mrs M., *A Modern Herbal* Vols I and II, (Penguin Books).
Griggs, Barbara, *The Green Pharmacy* (Norman & Hobhouse, 1981).
Hoffmann, David, *Herbal Stress Control* (Thorsons, 1986).
Hoffmann, David, *The Herb User's Guide* (Thorsons, 1988).
Hoffmann, David, *The Holistic Herbal* (Element Books, 1983, new edn, 1990).

Lovelock, James, *GAIA: A New Look at Life on Earth* (Oxford University Press, 1979).

Lust, John, *The Herb Book* (Bantam Books, 1974).

Mabey R. and McIntyre M., *The New Herbalist* (Elm Tree, 1988).

McIntyre, Anne, *Herbs for Pregnancy and Childbirth* (Sheldon Press, 1988).

McIntyre, Michael, *Herbal Medicine for Everyone* (Penguin, 1989).

Mills, Simon, *Dictionary of Modern Herbalism* (Thorsons, 1987).

Mills, Simon (ed.), *Alternatives in Healing* (Macmillan, 1988).

Priest and Priest, *Herbal Medications* (L.N. Fowler & Co. Ltd., 1982).

Roberts, Frank, *Modern Herbalism for Digestive Disorders* (Thorsons, 1978).

Schultes and Hofmann, *Plants of the Gods* (Hutchinson Publishing Group, 1979).

Stuart, Malcom (ed.), *The Encyclopedia of Herbs and Herbalism* (Guild Publishing, 1986).

Tierra, Michael, *The Way of Herbs* (Orenda/Unity Press, 1980).

Trease and Evans, *Pharmacognosy* (13th edn, Baillere Tindall, 1989).

Weiss, Rudolf, *Herbal Medicine* (Beaconsfield Arcanum, 1988).

INDEX